Economics of Critical Care

Guest Editors

DONALD B. CHALFIN, MD, MS, FCCP, FCCM
JOHN A. RIZZO, PhD

CRITICAL CARE CLINICS

www.criticalcare.theclinics.com

Consulting Editor
RICHARD W. CARLSON, MD, PhD

January 2012 • Volume 28 • Number 1

SAUNDERS an imprint of ELSEVIER, Inc.

W.B. SAUNDERS COMPANY
A Division of Elsevier Inc.

Elsevier Inc. • 1600 John F. Kennedy Blvd., • Suite 1800 • Philadelphia, Pennsylvania 19103-2899

http://www.theclinics.com

CRITICAL CARE CLINICS Volume 28, Number 1
January 2012 ISSN 0749-0704, ISBN-13: 978-1-4557-3844-1

Editor: Patrick Manley

Critical Care Clinics (ISSN: 0749-0704) is published quarterly by Elsevier Inc., 360 Park Avenue South, New York, NY 10010-1710. Months of issue are January, April, July, and October. Business and Editorial Offices: 1600 John F. Kennedy Blvd., Suite 1800, Philadelphia, PA 19103-2899. Customer Service Office: 6277 Sea Harbor Drive, Orlando, FL 32887-4800. Periodicals postage paid at New York, NY and additional mailing offices. Subscription prices are $193.00 per year for US individuals, $463.00 per year for US institution, $94.00 per year for US students and residents, $238.00 per year for Canadian individuals, $574.00 per year for Canadian institutions, $278.00 per year for international individuals, $574.00 per year for international institutions and $137.00 per year for Canadian and foreign students/residents. To receive student/resident rate, orders must be accompanied by name of affiliated institution, date of term, and the signature of program/residency coordinator on institution letterhead. Orders will be billed at individual rate until proof of status is received. Foreign air speed delivery is included in all *Clinics* subscription prices. All prices are subject to change without notice. POSTMASTER: Send address changes to *Critical Care Clinics,* Elsevier Periodicals Customer Service, 11830 Westline Industrial Drive, St. Louis, MO 63146. **Customer Service: 1-800-654-2452 (US). From outside of the US, call 1-314-447-8871. Fax: 1-314-447-8029. E-mail: journalscustomerservice-usa@elsevier.com (for print support) or journalsonlinesupport-usa@elsevier.com (for online support).**

Reprints. For copies of 100 or more of articles in this publication, please contact the Commercial Reprints Department, Elsevier Inc., 360 Park Avenue South, New York, NY 10010-1710. Tel.: 212-633-3813; Fax: 212-462-1935; E-mail: reprints@elsevier.com.

Critical Care Clinics is also published in Spanish by Editorial Inter-Medica, Junin 917, 1er A, 1113, Buenos Aires, Argentina.

Critical Care Clinics is covered in *MEDLINE/PubMed (Index Medicus), EMBASE/Excerpta Medica, Current Concepts/Clinical Medicine, ISI/BIOMED, and Chemical Abstracts.*

Printed and bound by CPI Group (UK) Ltd, Croydon, CR0 4YY
Transferred to Digital Print 2012

Contributors

CONSULTING EDITOR

RICHARD W. CARLSON, MD, PhD
Chairman Emeritus, Department of Medicine, Maricopa Medical Center; Director, Medical Intensive Care Unit; Professor, University of Arizona College of Medicine; Professor, Department of Medicine, Mayo Graduate School of Medicine, Phoenix, Arizona

GUEST EDITORS

DONALD B. CHALFIN, MD, MS, FCCP, FCCM
Medical Director, Ibis Biosciences, Carlsbad, California

JOHN A. RIZZO, PhD
Professor of Economics and Preventive Medicine, Stony Brook University, Stony Brook, New York

AUTHORS

ANDREW N. CHALUPKA, BA
Medical Student, Harvard Medical School, Boston, Massachusetts

CHEE M. CHAN, MD, MPH
Pulmonary and Critical Care Medicine, Washington Hospital Center; Assistant Professor of Medicine, Georgetown University, Washington, DC

JIE CHEN, PhD
Assistant Professor of Economics, Department of Political Science, Economics, and Philosophy, City University of New York, College of Staten Island, Staten Island, New York

COLIN R. COOKE, MD, MSc
Division of Pulmonary & Critical Care Medicine, Center for Healthcare Outcomes & Policy, and Robert Wood Johnson Foundation Clinical Scholar Program, University of Michigan, Ann Arbor, Michigan

JUBRAN DAKWAR, MD
Fellow, Critical Care Medicine, Department of Anesthesiology and Critical Care Medicine, Memorial Sloan-Kettering Cancer Center, New York, New York

HAYLEY GERSHENGORN, MD
Assistant Professor, Division of Pulmonary, Critical Care, and Sleep Medicine, Albert Einstein College of Medicine, Beth Israel Medical Center, New York, New York

NEIL A. HALPERN, MD
Professor of Medicine and Anesthesiology, Weill Medical College of Cornell University; Chief, Critical Care Medicine Service, Department of Anesthesiology and Critical Care Medicine, Memorial Sloan-Kettering Cancer Center, New York, New York

ANTHONY H. HARRIS, MA, MSc
Professor and Deputy Director, Centre for Health Economics, Monash University, Melbourne, Australia

ALISA M. HIGGINS, MPH, BPhysio(Hons), Grad Dip Biostats
Research Fellow and PhD Scholar, Australian and New Zealand Intensive Care Research Centre, Department of Epidemiology and Preventive Medicine, School of Public Health and Preventive Medicine, Monash University, Melbourne, Australia

STEPHEN MUNN, MB, ChB, FACS, FRACS
Transplant Surgeon, New Zealand Liver Transplant Unit; Chair Clinical Practice Committee, Auckland District Health Board, Auckland, New Zealand

AMAY PARIKH, MD, MBA, MS
Columbia University Medical Center, New York, New York

STEPHEN M. PASTORES, MD
Professor of Medicine and Anesthesiology, Weill Medical College of Cornell University; Director, Critical Care Medicine Fellowship Program, Critical Care Medicine Service, Department of Anesthesiology and Critical Care Medicine, Memorial Sloan-Kettering Cancer Center, New York, New York

JOHN A. RIZZO, PhD
Professor of Economics and Preventive Medicine, Stony Brook University, Stony Brook, New York

DAMON C. SCALES, MD, PhD
Assistant Professor, Interdepartmental Division of Critical Care Medicine, University of Toronto; Department of Critical Care Medicine, Sunnybrook Health Sciences Centre, Toronto, Canada

ANDREW SHAW, MB, FRCA, FCCM
Duke University Medical Center, Durham, North Carolina

ANDREW F. SHORR, MD, MPH
Pulmonary and Critical Care Medicine, Washington Hospital Center; Association Professor of Medicine, Georgetown University, Washington, DC

STEPHEN STREAT, MB, ChB, FRACP
Intensivist, Department of Critical Care Medicine; Deputy Chair Clinical Practice Committee, Auckland District Health Board, Auckland, New Zealand

DANIEL TALMOR, MD, MPH
Vice Chair for Critical Care, Department of Anesthesia, Critical Care, and Pain Medicine, Beth Israel Deaconess Medical Center; Associate Professor of Anesthesia, Harvard Medical School, Boston, Massachusetts

HANNAH WUNSCH, MD, MSc
Assistant Professor of Anesthesiology and Epidemiology, Departments of Anesthesiology and Epidemiology, Columbia University, New York, New York

MARYA D. ZILBERBERG, MD, MPH
Adjunct Associate Professor of Biostatistics and Epidemiology, School of Public Health and Health Sciences, University of Massachusetts, Amherst; President & CEO, EviMed Research Group, LLC, Goshen, Massachusetts; Senior Fellow, Jefferson School of Population Health, Thomas Jefferson University, Philadelphia, Pennsylvania

Contents

Preface: Health Economics and Critical Care   ix

Donald B. Chalfin and John A. Rizzo

Costs of Critical Care Medicine   1

Stephen M. Pastores, Jubran Dakwar, and Neil A. Halpern

> The main drivers of critical care medicine (CCM) costs are the numbers and use of intensive care unit (ICU) beds. The Russell equation, an indirect costing methodology, is most commonly used to estimate national CCM costs. Calculating national CCM costs in a standardized manner remains challenging because there is no universal approach to defining the types of hospitals, ICU beds, days, and billing codes to be included in the overall cost. Although numerous CCM cost-containment strategies have been proposed or implemented, CCM cost reduction remains elusive, and measuring cost remains challenging, given the complexities involved in assessing costs.

Health Economic Methods: Cost-Minimization, Cost-Effectiveness, Cost-Utility, and Cost-Benefit Evaluations   11

Alisa M. Higgins and Anthony H. Harris

> Health care resources are limited, and health care providers must strive to maximize health benefits to patients within available resources. This is becoming increasingly important in critical care as demand for services grows and costs associated with treatment increase. Economic evaluations enable comparisons of both the costs and effects of an intervention. There are four main types: cost-minimization, cost-effectiveness, cost-utility, and cost-benefit. The costs associated with the intervention are measured in monetary units (dollars); the evaluation types differ with respect to how outcomes are measured. This article introduces the methodology for performing these economic evaluations, highlighting important aspects regarding critical care.

Economics of ICU Organization and Management   25

Hannah Wunsch, Hayley Gershengorn, and Damon C. Scales

> The intensive care unit (ICU) is a complex system and the economic implications of altering care patterns in the ICU can be difficult to unravel. Few studies have specifically examined the economics of implementing organizational and management changes or acknowledged the many competing economic interests of patient, hospital, payer, and society. With continuously increasing healthcare costs, there is a great need for more studies focused on the optimal organization of the ICU. These studies should not focus solely on reductions in ICU length of stay but should strive to measure the true costs of care within a given healthcare system.

Economics of Mechanical Ventilation and Respiratory Failure   39

Colin R. Cooke

For patients with acute respiratory failure, mechanical ventilation provides the most definitive life-sustaining therapy. Because of the intense resources required to care for these patients, its use accounts for considerable costs. There is great societal need to ensure that use of mechanical ventilation maximizes societal benefits while minimizing costs, and that mechanical ventilation, and ventilator support in general, is delivered in the most efficient and cost-effective manner. This review summarizes the economic aspects of mechanical ventilation and summarizes the existing literature that examines its economic impact cost effectiveness.

The Economics of Sepsis   57

Andrew N. Chalupka and Daniel Talmor

Sepsis, severe sepsis, and septic shock impose a growing economic burden on health care systems globally. This article first describes the epidemiology of sepsis within the United States and internationally. It then reviews costs associated with sepsis and its management in the United States and internationally, including general cost sources in intensive care, direct costs of sepsis, and indirect costs of the burden of illness imposed by sepsis. Finally, it examines the cost-effectiveness of sepsis interventions, focusing on formal cost-effectiveness analyses of nosocomial sepsis prevention strategies, drotrecogin alfa (activated), and integrated sepsis protocols.

The Economics of Cardiovascular Disease in the United States   77

Jie Chen and John A. Rizzo

Cardiovascular disease is the leading cause of death in the United States, and thus its clinical and economic implications are enormous. In an increasingly cost-conscious economic environment, it is important to understand not only the effectiveness of treatments and technologies but also their cost-effectiveness. The authors review and summarize the evidence on cost-effectiveness of surgical versus medical treatments. This evidence should prove useful at the patient bedside as well as assist policy makers and third party payers in deciding what treatments to cover.

Economic Aspects of Preventing Health Care–Associated Infections in the Intensive Care Unit   89

Marya D. Zilberberg and Andrew F. Shorr

Infection prevention is critical to providing a high standard of care in the intensive care unit (ICU). Recent focus on eliminating health care–associated infections (HAIs) has met with variable results. Although evidence-based as far as their components, policy-driven bundled HAI prevention interventions have been evaluated in a limited and potentially biased fashion for their effectiveness, and analyses of their cost-effectiveness are lacking. We use ventilator-associated pneumonia as the case study to illustrate the pitfalls and challenges of arriving at the optimal HAI preventive strategies in the ICU.

The Economics of Renal Failure and Kidney Disease in Critically Ill Patients   99

Amay Parikh and Andrew Shaw

The kidney is an organ of opportunity cost in the sense that its function is often sacrificed in exchange for the preservation of function of another organ, organ system, or multiorgan process. The ICU setting represents the intersection of multiple organ systems that may result in kidney disease. When the severity of acute kidney injury warrants consideration of renal replacement therapy (RRT), multiple modalities such as peritoneal dialysis, intermittent hemodialysis, and continuous RRT are considered. In this article, the economic issues germane to AKI and its treatment in the ICU setting are presented.

Economic and Outcomes Aspects of Venous Thromboembolic Disease   113

Chee M. Chan and Andrew F. Shorr

Critically ill patients clearly face an increased risk for developing venous thromboembolic disease (VTE). Upon admission, all critical care patients should be immediately assessed for and prescribed VTE prophylaxis as it can significantly reduce VTE occurrence, its potential sequelae, and costs associated with VTE treatment. The financial burden associated with VTE is substantial. Longer ICU and hospital lengths of stay, pharmacy costs, and further outpatient management all contribute considerably to the economic burden of disease. The importance of this healthcare issue should motivate hospital administrators and physicians to systematically initiate thromboprophylaxis in all ICU patients.

Health Economics and Health Technology Assessment: Perspectives from Australia and New Zealand   125

Stephen Streat and Stephen Munn

Formal health economics and health technology assessment (HTA) processes, including cost-effectiveness and cost-utility analysis, are variably used to inform decisions about public and private health service funding and service provision. In general, pharmaceuticals have been subject to more sophisticated health economic analyses and HTAs and for a longer time than either devices or procedures. HTA has been performed by a number of different entities. While HTA shares many common features across the world, its uses, approaches, applications, and impact differ throughout the world. This article will discuss some of the general attributes of HTA and will focus on its specific applications in Australia and New Zealand.

Index   135

FORTHCOMING ISSUES

April 2012

CPR
Wanchung Tang, MD, *Guest Editor*

July 2012

Toxicology
James Kruse, MD, *Guest Editor*

October 2012

Nonmalignant Hematology
Robert I. Parker, MD, *Guest Editor*

RECENT ISSUES

October 2011

Venous Thromboembolism in Critical Care
Kenneth E. Wood, DO, *Guest Editor*

July 2011

ALI and ARDS: Challenges and Advances
Krishnan Raghavendran, MD and
Lena M. Napolitano, MD, *Guest Editors*

April 2011

Biomarkers in the Critically Ill Patient
Mitchell M. Levy, MD, *Guest Editor*

THE CLINICS ARE NOW AVAILABLE ONLINE!

Access your subscription at:
www.theclinics.com

Preface

Health Economics and Critical Care

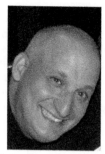 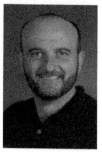

Donald B. Chalfin, MD, MS, FCCP, FCCM
Guest Editors

John A. Rizzo, PhD

Health care has always had to grapple with limited resources, but the challenge that society increasingly faces today is how to continue to deliver high-quality care that yields meaningful outcomes in the face of ever-constrained budgets. Perhaps this missive is most imperative in the critical care setting, where costs are disproportionately high relative to other medical services, and outcomes are usually the most tenuous, uncertain, and unpredictable. Inherent in all this is the notion that health care decisions should never be a matter of cutting costs or assessing the financial ramifications of a particular endeavor, but rather, a matter of allocating scare resources toward those services, programs, and interventions that will provide the greatest overall benefit to those in need. The operative word, then, is value and thus the task incumbent upon us all is how we assess, convey, promote, and even enhance value for our patients.

Health economic evaluations have increasingly appeared in the medical literature in general and in critical care medicine in particular but, more importantly, the critical care practitioner is increasingly called upon to participate in difficult decisions, both at the bedside and in the boardroom, that have vast health economic and clinical ramifications in terms of which services to provide, how one's unit should be staffed, and what is the overall benefit relative to the resources that are expended for a particular intervention. It is with this sentiment in mind that we devote this issue of *Critical Care Clinics* to health economics, in which a broad introduction of health economic methods are provided along with more detailed, specialty-based overviews of specific applications and implications, from sepsis to cardiovascular disease, to mechanical ventilation and respiratory care, to organizational issues in the ICU and so forth. We hope that from the following articles, the reader gets a sense of how economic questions are approached and how issues concerning cost, cost-effectiveness, and the determination of overall economic impact are addressed. For better

Crit Care Clin 28 (2012) ix–xi
doi:10.1016/j.ccc.2011.10.015
0749-0704/12/$ – see front matter © 2012 Elsevier Inc. All rights reserved.

criticalcare.theclinics.com

or worse, intensivists and all ICU professionals will likely have to "weigh in" on issues, initiatives, and programs that require an understanding of value, cost, and economic impact and we hope that the work in this edition provides a sense of how indeed "value" may be quantified and maximized so that all patients who require critical care services stand the greatest chance to benefit from our expertise.

We are fortunate to have the "editorial erudition" from many experts from all over, who all took the time from their hectic routines to research their topics and contribute to this edition. It is always a privilege and a joy to work with such fine and dedicated individuals and to learn not only from their submissions but also from their often unique perspectives as to how economic methods should be applied, interpreted, and even enacted. To them, and to Patrick Manley at Elsevier, who always worked to ensure that deadlines were met in order to produce a high-quality product, we owe our deepest thanks and warmest gratitude.

Donald B. Chalfin, MD, MS, FCCP, FCCM
Ibis Biosciences
Carlsbad, CA, USA

John A. Rizzo, PhD
Department of Economics
Stony Brook University
N-637 Social and Behavioral Sciences Building
Stony Brook, NY 11794, USA

E-mail addresses:
dbchalfin@gmail.com (D.B. Chalfin)
rizzologic@gmail.com (J.A. Rizzo)

Dedication

To Greg, whose wit, energy, intellect, drive, and charm always remind me that he is not just my son but also my greatest teacher and most inspiring hero.

&

To Lynn, my wife, my partner, my inspiration, my love, and the source of so much of my newfound joy, who has not only rekindled my smile and broadened my life with her two very special "Isagirls," but who has also shown me that there is truly a way forward . . . and beyond.

Eu te amo, para sempre e sempre

DBC

To my wife, Carmela
JAR

Costs of Critical Care Medicine

Stephen M. Pastores, MD[a,b,*], Jubran Dakwar, MD[b],
Neil A. Halpern, MD[b]

KEYWORDS

- Costs • Critical care medicine • Intensive care
- Economics • Russell equation • Cost control

"By a wide margin the biggest threat to our nation's balance sheet is the skyrocketing cost of health care." —*President Barack Obama, March 2009*

Health care in the United States is by far the most expensive in the world. In 2009, national health expenditures (NHE) in the United States were estimated to be $2.5 trillion accounting for 17.6% of the gross domestic product (GDP).[1] Although landmark legislation and governmental programs have recently been passed and initiated with a focus toward cost control,[2,3] the US patient care delivery system has been continuously evolving over the last 20 years. Acute care hospitals have closed, and inpatient care has shifted to the outpatient arena. Concomitantly, the number of critical care medicine (CCM) beds has steadily increased as hospitalized patients are sicker. With the escalating scrutiny of health care resources, the high costs associated with CCM have become a serious national concern. In 2005, CCM costs in the United States were estimated to be $81.7 billion, accounting for 13.4% of hospital costs, 4.1% of the NHE, and 0.66% of the GDP.[4]

Understanding how CCM costs are determined is crucial to informing our policy decisions and guiding cost reduction strategies.[5] The 2 main drivers of CCM costs are the number of intensive care unit (ICU) beds and their utilization. The United States appears to devote more of its hospital resources to CCM than other countries. This is evidenced by the United States having among the highest ICU-bed-to-population (20 ICU beds per 100,000) and ICU-to-hospital-bed (9 per 100 hospital beds) ratios in the world.[6] The United States also applies far more CCM services for medical patients, the elderly, and at the end of life than other developed countries.[7,8]

The authors have nothing to disclose.

[a] Department of Medicine and Anesthesiology, Weill Medical College of Cornell University, New York, NY, USA

[b] Department of Anesthesiology and Critical Care Medicine, Memorial Sloan-Kettering Cancer Center, 1275 York Avenue C-1179, New York, NY 10065, USA

* Corresponding author. Department of Anesthesiology and Critical Care Medicine, Weill Medical College of Cornell University, 1275 York Avenue C-1179, New York, NY 10065.

E-mail address: pastores@mskcc.org

Crit Care Clin 28 (2012) 1–10

doi:10.1016/j.ccc.2011.10.003

0749-0704/12/$ – see front matter © 2012 Elsevier Inc. All rights reserved.

criticalcare.theclinics.com

Table 1		
National hospital and billing databases: ICU bed and day data		
Database	**Data Source**	**Beds, Days, and Cost Data**
AHA Hospital Statistics produced by the American Hospital Association (AHA)	Annual AHA surveys voluntarily submitted by hospitals	ICU beds by ICU type and units Adjusted expenses per inpatient day (see **Fig. 1**)
Healthcare Cost Report Information System (HCRIS) produced by the Centers for Medicare and Medicaid Services (CMS)	Annual Hospital Cost Reports completed by each hospital (nonfederal) and submitted to CMS	ICU bed and days by ICU type (see **Fig. 1**) ICU days for Medicare and Medicaid Hotel type costs attributed to ICU days
Medicare Provider and Review File (MedPAR) produced by the Centers for Medicare and Medicaid Services (CMS)	Compilation of Medicare beneficiary hospital bills	Hospital and ICU days Hospital and ICU day room and board charges for Medicare beneficiaries

The AHA publications have not published ICU bed data since 1994; ICU bed data may be obtained through direct requests to the AHA Health Forum group. Likewise, HCRIS requires purchase of the HCRIS dataset, and analysis requires experts familiar with the HCRIS data layout and governmental rules.

NATIONAL HOSPITAL DATABASES AND CCM DATA

There are two national US databases that track hospital use and cost data (**Table 1**). The first is the commercially available Hospital Statistics report that is annually published by the American Hospital Association (AHA).[9] This dataset contains information obtained from the yearly AHA surveys that are voluntarily completed by almost all US hospitals. The second is the Healthcare Cost Report Information System (HCRIS), a dataset composed of the Hospital Cost Reports that are annually submitted by all nonfederal hospitals. HCRIS is maintained by the Centers for Medicare and Medicaid Services (CMS).[10]

The AHA reports and HCRIS contain ICU bed data focusing primarily on the number of ICU beds. The 2 datasets, however, differ in their ICU bed type classifications and bed totals, thus limiting their comparability (**Tables 2** and **3**). Additionally, the AHA publishes estimates of the number of ICUs by type but has no data on ICU bed use; in contrast, HCRIS does not track the number of ICUs, but does include ICU utilization (days) by ICU bed type. HCRIS also identifies ICU days for all inpatients and specifically for the Medicare and Medicaid subgroups.[4] With regard to costs, the AHA has hospital and inpatient cost data, but none specific to critical care. By comparison, HCRIS has ICU cost data, but these costs are limited to room and board type expenditures and do not include all the other expenses (eg, nursing, medications, imaging, laboratory) associated with an ICU stay.

Medicare beneficiary use of critical care can also be determined from the Medicare Provider Analysis and Review (MedPAR) File (see **Table 1**).[11] MedPAR, a hospital claims CMS dataset, tracks ICU use (days) and costs (room and board charges) by specific ICU billing revenue codes (**Table 4**). However, MedPAR, like HCRIS, cannot be used to calculate a comprehensive ICU cost per day.

ICU Types	HCRIS	AHA
Table 2		
Comparison of ICU bed types between the HCRIS[10] and the AHA datasets[9]		
Intensive care	X	
Medical-surgical		X
Coronary/cardiac care	X	X
Surgical	X	
Burn	X	X
Premature	X[a]	
Neonatal	X[a]	X
Pediatric	X[a]	X
Psychiatric	X[a]	
Detoxification	X[a]	
Trauma	X[a]	
Other intensive care		X
Other Special Care	X[a]	X[b]

Intensive care is the general ICU category in HCRIS; Medical-surgical is the general ICU category in the AHA. Both HCRIS and AHA share similar coronary/cardiac, burn, neonatal and pediatric ICU categories. Unlike HCRIS, the AHA does not have a distinct surgical ICU category; instead, surgical ICU beds may either be included in medical-surgical or the other intensive care categories. For reporting purposes in the past, the AHA bundled the "other intensive care" beds within the medical-surgical ICU category. Both HCRIS and AHA have a category called o*ther special care.*

[a] In HCRIS, "other special care" includes 6 ICU types (premature, neonatal, pediatric, psychiatric, detoxification, and trauma); these can be bundled together as "other special care" or reported individually.

[b] In contrast, within the AHA, the "other special care" category may represent step-down beds, but it is poorly defined and is reported as a stand-alone, non-ICU category.

CRITICAL CARE COST CALCULATIONS IN THE UNITED STATES

The main tenets for understanding CCM utilization and cost in the United States were outlined in 1984 by Berenson[12] in a report commissioned by the US government. Recognizing the limitations of the national hospital databases, Berenson suggested that the Russell equation, first described in 1979, be used to "indirectly" calculate national CCM costs.[12,13]

The primary goal of the Russell equation is to establish an all-inclusive average ICU cost per day (**Fig. 1**, step 1). This value is then multiplied by the number of ICU days per year to determine the national US CCM cost (**Fig. 1**, step 2). The Russell equation relies on various data sources for costs and bed days (see **Table 1**). The *adjusted expenses per inpatient day,* as determined annually by the AHA, is commonly used as the cost basis for the Russell equation.[9] In the first iteration of Russell equation based CCM cost studies,[14,15] hospital days were obtained directly from the AHA dataset; however, ICU and non-ICU days were estimated.[14,15] Contemporary CCM cost studies obtain hospital, ICU, and non-ICU days directly from HCRIS.[4,16–18] The most intriguing component of the Russell equation is the ratio of ICU/non-ICU costs per day.[12–15]

SUMMARY OF US ICU COST STUDIES

Berenson[12] estimated that $13 to $15 billion was spent for the care of adult critically ill and coronary care patients in 1982. This CCM cost represented 14% to 17% of

Step 1:

Adjusted expenses per inpatient day =

$$\frac{([\text{non-ICU inpatient days}][\text{non-ICU cost per day}]) + ([\text{ICU inpatient days}][\textbf{\textit{ICU cost per day}}])}{\text{Hospital inpatient days}}$$

Step 2: ***ICU cost per day*** x ICU days = national CCM costs

Fig. 1. The Russell equation. The "adjusted expenses per inpatient day" is obtained from the AHA Hospital Statistics reports. This value is an average cost per inpatient day across all hospital bed types including ICU and non-ICU days. In the early Russell equation studies, inpatient days were obtained from the AHA; ICU days were estimated (ICU days = ICU beds [AHA source] × 365 days × ICU occupancy rate [84%]),[14,15] and then non-ICU days were determined as the difference between hospital and ICU days. More contemporaneously, ICU and non-ICU days are taken directly from the HCRIS dataset.[4,16–18] When solving the equation, the ICU *cost per day* equals (non-ICU cost per day) × (ICU/non-ICU cost ratio). This ratio is commonly accepted to be 3:1. Thus, for our purposes, the cost of an ICU day is 3 times that of a non-ICU day.

total inpatient community hospital costs and 0.7% of the GDP. Using the Russell equation, Jacobs and Noseworthy, estimated 1986 ICU costs in the United States at $33.9 billion, approximating 20% of all inpatient hospital costs, and 0.7% of the GDP (**Table 5**).[14] Halpern and coworkers[15] estimated US CCM costs to be $29.5 billion in 1986 (0.7% of GDP) and $55 billion (0.9% of GDP) in 1992 when they similarly solved the Russell equation. These latter two CCM cost studies used a 3:1 ICU/non-ICU cost ratio and formed the basis for the general perception that CCM costs approximate 1% of the GDP.

Subsequently, with the shift from estimates of ICU days to their direct measurement from HCRIS, the recalculated CCM costs were found to be much lower than previously thought for comparable years.[4,16] For example, the total CCM cost in 1986 was $21.2 billion (0.48% of GDP)[16] rather than the earlier documented $33.9 billion (0.7% of GDP)[14] and $29.5 billion (0.7% of GDP)[15] (see **Table 5**). Likewise, in 1992, the CCM cost was $38.9 billion (0.62% of GDP) rather than $55 billion (0.9% of GDP). We have ascribed the decreased CCM costs to our solving the Russell equation with actual and annual "CCM inpatient days" data that were lower than those directly and intermittently determined estimates formerly used[16] (see **Table 5**). Additionally, the earlier CCM cost studies did not specify the number and type (all hospitals vs short-term, nonfederal, general) of hospitals being studied. Presently, well-defined groups of acute care hospitals with ICU beds are consistently analyzed. Finally, the cost basis of the early Russell equation studies may have included both outpatient and inpatient costs rather than inpatient costs alone, thus artificially increasing the ICU cost per day.

Contemporary analyses show that CCM costs were $56.6 billion (0.58% of GDP) in 2000 and $81.7 billion (0.66% of GDP) in 2005,[4] clearly indicating that annual CCM costs are less than 1% of the GDP.[4,15,16] Although CCM may appear to incur less cost than perceived in the past, it is possible that the current "data"-driven approach to the Russell equation underestimates CCM costs. The AHA-adjusted expenses per inpatient day determination does not take into account all inpatient costs, because the private billings of physicians are not included. The ICU days from HCRIS may not reflect all ICU care in a hospital because HCRIS does not track ICU-level care rendered in non-ICU settings (ie, Emergency Department, Post-Anesthesiology Care

Table 3
Comparison of ICU bed totals by ICU type for 2005: HCRIS[4] and the AHA datasets

Intensive Care Unit Types	HCRIS	AHA
Intensive care	55,996	
Medical-surgical		39,306
Coronary/cardiac care	11,757	14,581
Surgical	4525	
Burn	1194	1222
Premature	190	
Neonatal	15,127	17,113
Pediatric	1924	3909
Psychiatric	353	
Detoxification	1761	
Trauma	1128	
Other intensive care		5545
Other special care	—[a]	17,422[b]
ICU beds-total	93,955	81,670
Hospital bed-total	633,998	633,556
Hospitals reporting ICU beds	3150[c]	3090[d]

AHA data source: AHA Annual Survey Database, FY2005. Chicago: Health Forum LLC, an American Hospital Association company, 2006.

[a] HCRIS: "other special care" includes premature, neonatal, pediatric, psychiatric, detoxification, and trauma ICU types.

[b] AHA: "other special care" includes step-down beds and are not included in the ICU bed total.

[c] HCRIS: Acute care (short term, general and specialty care, and childrens and pediatrics) hospitals.

[d] AHA: Total community hospitals.

Unit). The recent HCRIS-based studies did not include all ICU beds in the United States because ICU care rendered in federal and less acute hospitals was excluded.[4,16]

ALTERNATIVE USES AND APPROACHES TO SOLVING THE RUSSELL EQUATION

Beyond determining national CCM costs, the Russell equation methodology has also been applied to defined hospital networks[15] and populations.[19,20] In these analyses, all data to solve the Russell equation was obtained from network or population-specific datasets rather than the AHA or HCRIS. Halpern and colleagues[15] determined ICU cost per day for Department of Veterans Affairs (DVA) medical centers (1986 to 1992) either directly from the DVA Cost Distribution Report (CDR) or through the Russell equation using cost and use data from the CDR. ICU costs per day were noted to be comparable when the 3:1 ICU/non-ICU cost ratio was used to solve the Russell equation. In the ensuing decade, Cooper and Linde-Zwirble[19] and Milbrandt and coworkers[20] examined ICU costs specifically for Medicare beneficiaries using the MedPAR file and the Russell equation. These investigators found that a 2:1 ICU/non-ICU cost ratio is more appropriate than the 3:1 value used historically. They ascribed the decrease in the ratio to an increase in the average cost of a ward day that is not matched by a similar increase in the cost of an ICU day. If the global US CCM cost would be recalculated using the lower (2:1) ratio to solve the Russell equation, then the average cost of an ICU day would be even less than current estimates. For

Table 4
Critical care bed categories and individual billing (revenue) codes: HCRIS versus MedPAR

HCRIS (Cost Centers)	MedPAR Categories	Billing (Revenue) Codes (0200–0219)	
ICU	Intensive care[b]	ICU: general classification	0200
Surgical ICU		ICU: surgical	0201
		ICU: medical	0202
		ICU: pediatrics	0203
		ICU: psychiatric	0204
		ICU: *post/intermediate*	0206
Burn ICU		ICU: burn care	0207
		ICU: trauma	0208
Other special care[a]		ICU: other	0209
Coronary care unit (CCU)	Coronary care[c]	CCU: general classification	0210
		CCU: myocardial infarction	0211
		CCU: pulmonary care	0212
		CCU: heart transplant	0213
		CCU: *post/intermediate*	0214
		CCU: other	0219

Both the intensive care and coronary care groups of MedPAR include the post/intermediate codes (0206 and 0214), which may reflect step-down days. Revenue Codes 0205 and 0215– 0218 are reserved for future use.

[a] "Other special care" includes premature, neonatal, pediatrics, psychiatric, detoxification, and trauma.

[b] "Intensive care" contains aggregate data from Intensive Care (ICU) Revenue Codes 0200–0209.

[c] "Coronary care" contains aggregate data from Coronary Care (CCU) Revenue Codes 0210–0219.

example, using the lower ratio, the ICU cost per day was calculated at $2,462 in 2000[19] and $2,575 per day in 2004,[20] values lower than the costs previously calculated for similar years (see **Table 5**).

Although the ICU cost per day may be lower upon recalculation with the lower ICU/non-ICU cost ratio, the annual CCM cost rests primarily on the number of ICU days used in a given year. This is true whether the costs are being determined nationally or for a defined hospital network or population. However, even determining the number of ICU days may be challenging. A recent retrospective analysis comparing Medicare ICU days in HCRIS and MedPAR in all US nonfederal hospitals showed consistent and large discrepancies between the 2 datasets.[18] These differences were attributed to anomalies between CCM cost center codes in HCRIS and revenue and billing codes in MedPAR (see **Table 4**). At first glance, the HCRIS and MedPAR CCM bed type codes appear to be fairly straightforward. However, MedPAR researchers primarily used two broad critical care categories: intensive care (9 ICU codes) and coronary care unit (6 CCU codes) (see **Table 4**), rather than individual ICU and CCU billing codes. Investigators did not recognize that MedPAR was bundling "post/intermediate" ICU and CCU codes into the large intensive and coronary care categories. The post/intermediate codes may represent step-down type days and not actual ICU or CCU days. Thus, the intensive and coronary care day counts in MedPAR were artificially increased, generating the disparities in ICU and CCU days observed between HCRIS and MedPAR. These database differences point to the well-known

Table 5
US intensive care unit beds, days and costs: 1986–2005

Study Year (References)	ICU Beds (Thousands)	ICU Beds Source	ICU Cost Per Day ($, Thousands)	ICU Days (Million)	ICU Days Source	ICU Cost Per Year ($, Billion)	CCM % of Hospital Costs	CCM % of GDP
Comparison of 1986 bed and cost data								
1986[14]	85.0	AHA	1296	26.1	Estimate[a]	33.9	20	0.7
1986[15]	85.3	AHA	1130	26.1	Estimate[a]	29.5	18	0.7
1986[16]	70.2	HCRIS	1277	16.6	HCRIS	21.2	11.8	0.48
Comparison of 1992 bed and cost data								
1992[15]	96.7	AHA	1857	29.6	Estimate[a]	55	20	0.9
1992[16]	79.4	HCRIS	2005	19.4	HCRIS	38.9	12.7	0.62
2000 and 2005 bed and cost data								
2000[4]	88.2	HCRIS	2698	21	HCRIS	56.6	13.6	0.58
2005[4]	93.9	HCRIS	3518	23.2	HCRIS	81.7	13.4	0.66

All dollars are expressed as "current" dollars and are not indexed.
[a] Calculated CCM days = ICU beds × 365 days × ICU occupancy rate. ICU beds were taken from AHA and the ICU occupancy rate used was 84%.[14,15]

but unavoidable vagaries and inconsistencies observed when analyzing and comparing large databases[21,22] and highlight the need for researchers to carefully determine when an ICU day is truly an ICU day.

While HCRIS tracks Medicaid CCM use in a limited manner,[4] to date, CMS does not maintain a global Medicaid dataset comparable to the national inclusivity of Medicare data in MedPAR. This deficiency exists because Medicaid is dually managed by the federal and state governments, whereas Medicare is predominantly federally administered. The lack of such a Medicaid database may limit our understanding of the potential expansion in CCM use over the next decade as uninsured persons are added to the ranks of Medicaid as a result of the recently passed government health care bill.[23,24]

LIMITATIONS OF GLOBAL ICU COST APPROACHES

The CCM costing approaches discussed here focus on average daily and aggregate yearly CCM costs of care. Costs attributable to components of CCM care (staffing, technology, medications, and patient care) are not identified. The Russell equation approach also may give the impression that all ICU days are similar in cost. This, however, is not true, as the first day of ICU care is far more resource intensive than subsequent days.[25,26] Additionally, the average ICU daily cost may vary based on ICU type.

COST CONTROL STRATEGIES

Given the high costs associated with CCM, cost control strategies have been proposed or implemented by clinicians, hospital administrators, and policy makers.[27] These strategies include rationing care,[28] reducing unnecessary variation in care by regionalization of critical care services,[29,30] caring for critically ill patients in non-ICU settings (telemetry, step-down units, postanesthesia care units, and ventilator units), fast-tracking surgical patients,[31] providing telemedicine coverage to ICUs to enhance safety and efficacy,[32–34] using nonphysician providers in the ICU,[35] and implementing care bundles, protocols and guidelines.[36,37] It may be quite difficult to discern whether CCM costs can actually be reduced regardless of the method of cost determination or the strategy of cost reduction used. Cost containment approaches all seem promising at the outset, but they may simply shift costs from the ICU to other cost centers, creating an illusion of CCM cost reduction.

SUMMARY

Critical care medicine is expensive and continues to grow in a shrinking US hospital system. The main drivers of CCM costs are the numbers and use of ICU beds. Existing hospital databases do not contain all the requisite elements to directly measure CCM costs. Therefore, the Russell equation, an indirect costing methodology, is most commonly used to estimate national CCM costs. Calculating national CCM costs in a standardized manner remains challenging because there is no universal approach to defining the types of hospitals and ICU beds, days, and billing codes to be included in the overall cost. Recent studies clearly indicate that annual CCM costs account for less than 1% of the GDP. While numerous CCM cost-containment strategies have been proposed or implemented, CCM cost reduction remains elusive, and perhaps unattainable, given the complexities involved in assessing costs.

REFERENCES

1. NHE Fact Sheet. Available at: https://www.cms.gov/NationalHealthExpendData/25_NHE_Fact_Sheet.asp#TopOfPage. Accessed June 23, 2011.
2. Patient Protection and Affordable Care Act, Pub. L. No. 111–148, §10409, 124 Stat. 119, 978, 2010.
3. http://www.healthcare.gov/news/factsheets/partnership04122011a.html. Accessed June 23, 2011.
4. Halpern NA, Pastores SM. Critical care medicine in the United States 2000–2005: an analysis of bed numbers, occupancy rates, payer mix, and costs. Crit Care Med 2010;38(1):65–71.
5. Adhikari NK, Fowler RA, Bhagwanjee S, et al. Critical care and the global burden of critical illness in adults. Lancet 2010;376(9749):1339–46.
6. Wunsch H, Angus DC, Harrison DA, et al. Variation in critical care services across North America and Western Europe. Crit Care Med 2008;36(10):2787–93, e2781–2789.
7. Wunsch H, Linde-Zwirble WT, Harrison DA, et al. Use of intensive care services during terminal hospitalizations in England and the United States. Am J Respir Crit Care Med 2009;180(9):875–80.
8. Wunsch H, Angus DC, Harrison DA, et al. Comparison of medical admissions to intensive care units in the United States and United kingdom. Am J Respir Crit Care Med 2011;183(12):1666–73.
9. Fast Facts on US Hospitals Available at: http://www.aha.org/aha/resource-center/Statistics-and-Studies/fast-facts.html. Accessed June 23, 2011.
10. Hospital Cost Report. Available at: http://www.cms.gov/CostReports/02_Hospital CostReport.asp#TopOfPage. Accessed June 23, 2011.
11. MEDPAR Limited Data Set (LDS)—Hospital (National). Available at: http://www.cms.gov/LimitedDataSets/02_MEDPARLDSHospitalNational.asp TopOfPage. Accessed June 23, 2011.
12. Berenson RA. Intensive care units: costs, outcomes and decision making. Washington, DC: US Congress, Office of Technology Assessment; 1984.
13. Russell LB. Intensive care. technology in hospitals, medical advances and their diffusion. Washington, DC: The Brookings Institution; 1979. p. 41–70.
14. Jacobs P, Noseworthy TW. National estimates of intensive care utilization and costs: Canada and the United States. Crit Care Med 1990;18(11):1282–6.
15. Halpern NA, Bettes L, Greenstein R. Federal and nationwide intensive care units and healthcare costs: 1986–1992. Crit Care Med 1994;22(12):2001–7.
16. Halpern NA, Pastores SM, Greenstein RJ. Critical care medicine in the United States 1985–2000: an analysis of bed numbers, use, and costs. Crit Care Med 2004;32(6):1254–9.
17. Halpern NA, Pastores SM, Thaler HT, et al. Changes in critical care beds and occupancy in the United States 1985–2000: differences attributable to hospital size. Crit Care Med 2006;34(8):2105–12.
18. Halpern NA, Pastores SM, Thaler HT, et al. Critical care medicine use and cost among Medicare beneficiaries 1995–2000: major discrepancies between two United States federal Medicare databases. Crit Care Med 2007;35(3):692–9.
19. Cooper LM, Linde-Zwirble WT. Medicare intensive care unit use: analysis of incidence, cost, and payment. Crit Care Med 2004;32(11):2247–53.
20. Milbrandt EB, Kersten A, Rahim MT, et al. Growth of intensive care unit resource use and its estimated cost in Medicare. Crit Care Med 2008;36(9):2504–10.

21. Belzberg H, Murray J, Shoemaker WC, et al. Use of large databases for resolving critical care problems. New Horiz 1996;4(4):532–40.

22. Pronovost P, Angus DC. Using large-scale databases to measure outcomes in critical care. Crit Care Clin 1999;15(3):615–31, vii–viii.

23. Sparer M. Medicaid and the U.S. path to national health insurance. N Engl J Med 2009;360(4):323–5.

24. Wilson JF. Will all health care reform lead back to Medicaid? Ann Intern Med 2009;150(2):149–51.

25. Rapoport J, Teres D, Zhao Y, et al. Length of stay data as a guide to hospital economic performance for ICU patients. Med Care 2003;41(3):386–97.

26. Dasta JF, McLaughlin TP, Mody SH, et al. Daily cost of an intensive care unit day: the contribution of mechanical ventilation. Crit Care Med 2005;33(6):1266–71.

27. Halpern NA. Can the costs of critical care be controlled? Curr Opin Crit Care 2009;15(6):591–6.

28. Sinuff T, Kahnamoui K, Cook DJ, et al. Rationing critical care beds: a systematic review. Crit Care Med 2004;32(7):1588–97.

29. Garland A, Shaman Z, Baron J, et al. Physician-attributable differences in intensive care unit costs: a single-center study. Am J Respir Crit Care Med 2006;174(11): 1206–10.

30. Sinuff T, Adhikari NK, Cook DJ, et al. Mortality predictions in the intensive care unit: comparing physicians with scoring systems. Crit Care Med 2006;34(3):878–85.

31. Flynn M, Reddy S, Shepherd W, et al. Fast-tracking revisited: routine cardiac surgical patients need minimal intensive care. Eur J Cardiothorac Surg 2004;25(1):116–22.

32. Cummings J, Krsek C, Vermoch K, et al. Intensive care unit telemedicine: review and consensus recommendations. Am J Med Qual 2007;22:239–50.

33. Lilly CM, Cody S, Zhao H, et al. Hospital mortality, length of stay, and preventable complications among critically ill patients before and after tele-ICU reengineering of critical care processes. JAMA 2011;305(21):2175–83.

34. Morrison JL, Cai Q, Davis N, et al. Clinical and economic outcomes of the electronic intensive care unit: results from two community hospitals. Crit Care Med 2010;38(1):2–8.

35. Kleinpell RM, Ely EW, Grabenkort R. Nurse practitioners and physician assistants in the intensive care unit: an evidence-based review. Crit Care Med 2008;36(10): 2888–97.

36. Levy MM, Dellinger RP, Townsend SR, et al. The Surviving Sepsis Campaign: results of an international guideline-based performance improvement program targeting severe sepsis. Crit Care Med 2010;38(2):367–74.

37. Schramm GE, Kashyap R, Mullon JJ, et al. Septic shock: a multidisciplinary response team and weekly feedback to clinicians improve the process of care and mortality. Crit Care Med 2011;39(2):252–8.

Health Economic Methods: Cost-Minimization, Cost-Effectiveness, Cost-Utility, and Cost-Benefit Evaluations

Alisa M. Higgins, MPH, BPhysio(Hons), Grad Dip Biostats[a],*, Anthony H. Harris, MA, MSc[b]

KEYWORDS
- Economic evaluations • Cost-effectiveness • Costs
- Critical care

Resources in the health care system are limited, and it is important to maximize the health benefits to patients within the resources available. In the critical care setting, this is becoming increasingly important as the demand for services grows and the costs associated with treatment increase. In the United States, intensive care units (ICUs) consume more than 20% of total hospital costs despite accounting for only 10% of hospital beds.[1] As a result, economic evaluations are becoming increasingly important in guiding decision making in the critical care setting.

Economic evaluations involve the measurement of costs for two (or more) alternative interventions, the determination of the benefits associated with the interventions, and the subsequent combination of these costs and benefits. The assessment of both costs and benefits enables a more complete consideration of the "value" of an intervention—what additional benefit is provided for what additional cost. Economic evaluations aid health care professionals and decision makers to decide between competing alternative interventions within the critical care setting itself, and also facilitate funding decisions for critical care services, compared to allocating resources elsewhere in the health system.

There are four main types of economic evaluations: cost-minimization, cost-effectiveness, cost-utility, and cost-benefit (**Table 1**). In each type of evaluation, the

Alisa Higgins is supported by an NHMRC Public Health Scholarship (no. 579709).
The authors having nothing further to disclose.
[a] Australian and New Zealand Intensive Care Research Centre, Department of Epidemiology and Preventive Medicine, School of Public Health and Preventive Medicine, Monash University, 99 Commercial Road, Melbourne 3004, Australia
[b] Centre for Health Economics, Monash University, Melbourne 3800, Australia
* Corresponding author.
E-mail address: lisa.higgins@monash.edu

Crit Care Clin 28 (2012) 11–24
doi:10.1016/j.ccc.2011.10.002
0749-0704/12/$ – see front matter © 2012 Elsevier Inc. All rights reserved.

criticalcare.theclinics.com

Table 1
Comparison of different types of economic evaluations

Type of Evaluation	Measurement of Costs	Measurement of Benefits	Summary Measure
Cost-minimization analysis	Dollars	None	Dollars (difference in cost between alternatives)
Cost-effectiveness analysis	Dollars	Natural units/clinical outcome (eg, life-years gained, cases of ventilator-acquired pneumonia avoided)	Cost-effectiveness ratio (eg, dollars per life year gained)
Cost-utility analysis	Dollars	Healthy years or QALYs	Cost-utility ratio (eg, cost per QALY)
Cost-benefit analysis	Dollars	Dollars	Net gain or loss in dollars

costs associated with the intervention are measured in monetary units (dollars); the evaluation types differ with respect to how outcomes are measured. As many published economic evaluations in critical care have been found to be of poor quality,[2,3] it is essential that critical care clinicians understand the methodology for performing such evaluations, to enable them to appraise the available evidence critically and incorporate the recommendations into their practice as appropriate.[4] This article introduces the methodology for performing economic evaluations, highlighting important aspects with regard to critical care.

TYPES OF ECONOMIC EVALUATION
Cost-Minimization Analysis

Cost-minimization analyses measure the difference in costs between alternative interventions. When comparing the interventions, the assumption is made that the alternatives are equally effective, and therefore the difference is in costs only. The costs are compared, with the assumption that the intervention with the lower cost would be adopted.

Cost-Effectiveness Analysis

Cost-effectiveness analyses measure outcomes (effectiveness) in naturally occurring, health-related units, such as lives saved, life years gained, or cases of ventilator-acquired pneumonia prevented.[4] When the outcomes are combined with costs, a ratio (known as a cost-effectiveness ratio) of the net change in costs (between two interventions) divided by the net change in outcomes is produced. The net change in costs reflects the extra cost required to achieve the difference in outcome (such as life years gained), with the ratio expressed as the cost per outcome gained, such as the cost per life year gained or the cost per life saved. Cost-effectiveness analyses were recommended by the American Thoracic Society's workshop on outcome research as the primary method to measure the costs and effects of interventions in critical care.[5]

Cost-Utility Analysis

A specific type of cost-effectiveness analysis is a cost-utility analysis, in which benefits are measured in healthy year equivalents, which are most commonly expressed as quality-adjusted life-years (QALYs).[4] These combine mortality and morbidity into a single summary effectiveness measure.[6] QALYs are determined by multiplying the number of life-years gained by a utility, wherein a utility refers to the preferences individuals or society have for a particular set of health outcomes.[7] For example, an individual living for 2 years with a utility of 0.8 would have 1.6 QALYs. In general, utilities can range from 0 (equivalent to death) to 1 (equivalent to full health).[7] Although it is possible to determine utilities using direct methods such as the time trade-off or standard gamble, to date, economic evaluations in critical care have typically used indirect methods to determine utilities. The indirect methods involve responses to a quality of life (QOL) questionnaire being expressed as a utility using prescaled responses from a relevant reference group.[8] The two general and prefer-ence-based QOL questionnaires most commonly used and recommended for critical care are the SF-36 and EQ-5D.[9] Utilities can be derived directly from the EQ5D[10] or indirectly from the SF36.[11] Other questionnaires from which utilities can be derived include the 15D,[12] the HUI3,[13] and the AQoL.[14]

The advantage of cost-utility analyses is that they enable comparison of different interventions across numerous disease states to determine which interventions result in the greatest gain for a given expense. That is, the cost per QALY can be compared between, for example, the use of extracorporeal membrane oxygenation for acute respiratory distress syndrome and total hip replacements for osteoarthritis.

Cost-Benefit Analysis

In cost-benefit analyses, both costs and outcomes are measured in monetary units. When all outcomes have been valued in monetary terms, all of the costs are added up and subtracted from the dollar value of the outcomes. If the resulting total is positive, the outcomes outweigh the costs, and the intervention is favored. As with cost-utility analyses, the use of a common metric enables comparison between studies that evaluate different outcomes. The difficulty in performing cost-benefit analyses is in valuing the outcomes, such as extending life, in monetary terms. This is usually performed using either the human capital approach or the willingness to pay approach. The human capital approach values an improvement in health on the basis of future productive worth from being able to return to work.[8] The willingness to pay approach values an improvement in health on the basis of how much people are willing to pay for the improvement. There are concerns, however, that an individual's response in an interview may not reflect his or her actions in real life,[4] and therefore the values applied to a given outcome may not be accurate in a realistic clinical setting. Owing to the difficulties in valuing health outcomes, cost-benefit analyses are rarely used.

The descriptions of these economic evaluations show that they differ in aspects such as how benefits are valued. However, there are numerous methodology aspects that are common to all analyses, including the definition of perspective, the identifi-cation of alternatives, the determination of costs and outcomes, the combination of costs and outcomes, and sensitivity analyses to deal with uncertainty. The following sections outline each of these aspects, using early goal-directed therapy (EGDT) for severe sepsis as a working example.

ANALYSIS PERSPECTIVES

When conducting economic evaluations, it is necessary to define the perspective from which the evaluation is conducted. Perspectives can range from that of the patient to that of the ICU alone to a broader societal perspective. The perspective chosen impacts both which costs and which outcomes should be considered in the analysis. For example, if conducting an economic evaluation of EGDT from an ICU's perspective, only costs incurred by the ICU are included. Such costs may include personnel (medical, nursing, allied health), clinical support services (such as radiology and pathology), consumables (such as medications, clinical supplies, nonclinical supplies), and capital equipment costs. However, if conducting the analysis from a societal perspective, all costs (and benefits) should theoretically be included, regardless of who incurs the costs (or receives the benefits). Therefore, costs borne by patients and their relatives such as the costs of transport to health care appointments and lost wages should be included, as should the costs to the patient's employer as a result of the patient being absent from work.

Conducting analyses from a societal perspective is considered the gold standard, as it considers all potential costs and benefits of interest to society irrespective of who bears the costs or receives the benefits, and allows a comparison across all health interventions that compete for resources. The U.S. Public Health Service Panel on Cost-Effectiveness in Health and Medicine (PCEHM) recommends conducting a reference case from a societal perspective,[15] and the position statement of the American Thoracic Society (ATS) on Understanding Costs and Cost-Effectiveness in the Critically Ill concurs with this recommendation.[5] However, in a systematic review of the critical care cost-effectiveness literature, only 2 of 19 identified analyses conducted their evaluation from a societal perspective, with all others conducted from a health care perspective.[16] Conducting analyses from a societal perspective for critical care interventions can be difficult because they require a time horizon longer than that of most critical care studies, and as such, require data from multiple sources and numerous assumptions. As a result, the ATS position statement recognizes that there are instances in which conducting an evaluation from a provider perspective may be useful.[5]

IDENTIFYING ALTERNATIVES

The key economic efficiency question is how to allocate finite resources between alternative courses of action, and therefore economic evaluation involves comparing two or more interventions. In assessing any given intervention, its cost-effectiveness will differ depending on what it is compared with. Decision makers will be interested in the incremental costs and outcomes for a new intervention compared to current practice. Thus, it is commonly the case that the current standard of care is the comparator. Choosing the right alternative for the purposes of comparison is important. Comparing a new intervention to a costly or inefficient practice may artificially infer a new intervention is highly cost-effective. Likewise, comparing a new intervention to an out-of-date or little used intervention will not provide results that are generalizable to the broader population that may be the target of the intervention.

When appraising economic analyses to determine the applicability of results to the clinician's practice, the choice of comparator is an important consideration. For example, Pandharipande and colleagues compared the effects of dexmedetomidine with those of lorazepam for reducing the duration of delirium and coma in mechanically ventilated patients.[17] This comparison is no doubt highly informative in a treatment setting where lorazepam is a commonly used sedative in critical care. However, in countries such as Australia where lorazepam is not routinely used in critical care, the results would not be generalizable.

MEASURING COSTS

The true measure of the cost of a resource is what could have been achieved with that resource in its next best alternative use (known as opportunity cost).[5] In practice this is valued as the financial cost of the resource although there may be cases in which prices are distorted and this needs to be amended. Costs are typically measured using bottom-up microcosting methods, more aggregated bundled grouped costs such as diagnosis-related grouped costs, or charges.[4] Microcosting involves measuring the quantity of resources used for each patient and attaching a unit cost to each of the resources. Examples of resources include personnel (nursing, medical, allied health) time, medications, diagnostic tests, and transport costs. The resources used are often collected alongside clinical trials, or may be collected prospectively or retrospectively from patients' medical records (although this allows for collection of resources only from a provider perspective). Diagnosis-related grouping methods involve assigning a cost for similar types of patients (with respect to diagnosis). These costs are often available through health care provider accounting systems and take account of length of stay. Charges are values that use the market or administered price for treatment.[4] The use of charges is suboptimal, as they may not reflect actual costs and are very specific to given departments and institutions.[7] As charges do not reflect actual costs, a cost-to-charge index (which is publically available) is often used to adjust the charges; however, it is unclear what the resultant cost figure represents.[3] A large proportion of critical care economic evaluations to date have used charges (or adjusted charges) as a substitute for costs.[1]

Given the significant costs associated with critical care, it is essential that costs are captured appropriately in any economic evaluation. Costs will differ between patients depending on numerous factors including the diagnosis, the severity of illness, and the patient's age. Costs will also vary across health systems and countries,[4] and are affected by factors such as treatment patterns, treatment availability, physician preferences, and funding mechanisms. Further, as different methods exist to collect costs, comparing the results of different economic evaluations can be problematic. Ideally, a uniform approach to costing should be used to enable differences between groups or between studies to be due to patient, treatment, and unit characteristics, rather than due to a difference in costing methodology. At present, there is no standard approach to measuring costs. The ATS position statement recommends the most practical approach at this time is to estimate resource use and multiply this use by standard costs.[5]

In measuring costs it is necessary to determine which resources will be collected and this depends on the analysis perspective, the time horizon, and the resources which are expected to differ between groups in the economic evaluation. As economic evaluations compare the costs between two (or more) groups, costs that are common to both (or all) groups do not need to be measured. In addition, because of the effort required in collecting detailed resource use, items that are associated with minimal cost difference do not need to be collected in as much detail as high-cost items. Once resource use has been collected, a unit cost is required to convert resource use into a monetary measure.[3] Often, such unit costs are not readily available, and may differ between hospitals or regions (eg, the cost a hospital pays for a particular drug can vary between hospitals). As such, the unit cost used for each resource must be clearly stated in any economic evaluation.

MEASURING OUTCOMES

Outcomes in economic evaluations usually come from single studies or an overview of numerous studies. In using data estimates from single studies, such as a randomized controlled trial (RCT), it is important to recognize that trials are often performed under strict conditions and may not be typical of what would be expected under usual clinical conditions.[4] RCTs often include only very specific patients, may optimize treatment with the intervention, and carefully control other aspects of care. As such, the outcomes in an RCT may overestimate the treatment effect that would be expected in actual clinical practice.

A further problem for determining outcomes is that critical care trials often do not provide outcomes relevant for use in an economic evaluation. The PCEHM and ATS position statement both recommend using QALYs as the unit of effect in cost-effectiveness analyses; however, most critical care trials use measures of short-term (28-day or hospital) mortality as the primary endpoint.[18] The 2002 Brussels roundtable on "Surviving Intensive Care" recommended follow-up in critical care trials should be for at least 6 months and further recommended that the SF-36 and EQ-5D are the best suited instruments for measuring QOL.[9] Among critically ill patients, there is considerable mortality beyond hospital discharge,[9,19] and QOL remains diminished beyond discharge, with Timmers and colleagues having shown that QOL remains below population norms in surgical ICU patients more than 6 years after discharge.[20] Owing to the lack of long-term outcomes in current critical care trials, the outcomes required for economic evaluations often need to be obtained from other sources such as observational studies.

DISCOUNTING AND THE TIME HORIZON

Costs and benefits are time dependent and are rarely spent or accrued immediately.[6] We value a dollar more today than we would tomorrow given its capacity to earn interest. Discounting is the method used to value future costs and benefits in present-day value.[4] As a result, economic evaluations need to define the time period for which the analysis applies and discount costs and benefits to present values where the time periods exceeds 1 year. The time period chosen should be long enough to capture all of the differential effects of the different interventions.[8] There continues to be debate about what discount rate to use, with most recommendations varying between 3% and 6%.[8] The PCEHM and ATS position statement both recommend using a discount rate of 3%.[5,15]

COMBINING COSTS AND OUTCOMES

In all economic evaluations other than cost-minimization analyses, costs and outcomes are combined into a single metric for interpretation and comparative purposes. The metric in cost-benefit analyses is a monetary value, while cost-effectiveness and cost-utility analyses produce a cost-effectiveness ratio. This ratio provides a summary measure of the resources required to produce a particular level of health,[6] and is calculated as the difference in costs divided by the difference in benefits. In general, the lower the ratio, the better the gain derived for a given expenditure. That is, it costs less to generate a given unit of health outcome. The cost-effectiveness ratio can be plotted (with 95% confidence boundaries) on a cost-effectiveness plane (**Fig. 1**), which provides a graphical representation of cost-effectiveness. The plane can be considered to be in four sections. Interventions can be less effective and less costly (bottom left quadrant), more effective and more costly (top right quadrant), less effective and more costly (top left quadrant), or more effective and less costly (bottom right quadrant). Where the intervention is less effective and more costly, it clearly should not be implemented. Conversely, interventions that are more effective and less costly clearly should be implemented. Where an intervention is more effective and more costly or less effective and less costly, a decision needs to be made about what one is willing to pay to obtain an extra unit of effectiveness (or willing to save to lose a unit of effectiveness).

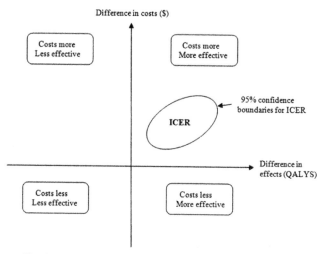

Fig. 1. The cost-effectiveness plane. ICER, incremental cost-effectiveness ratio. (*From* Higgins AM, Petilla V, Bellomo R, Harris AH, Nichol AD, Morrison SS. Expensive care—a rationale for economic evaluations in intensive care. Crit Care Resusc 2010;12:62–6; with permission.)

A decision on whether a therapy is cost-effective requires making a judgment about what society is willing to pay for a given outcome, such as life year gained. Typically, thresholds for cost-effectiveness exist (either implicit or explicit), where costs per outcome that are below the threshold are considered cost-effective (hence, the intervention is likely to be implemented), while those falling above the threshold are considered prohibitively expensive (and better use of funds exist). For example, if $100,000 per life year is the threshold, then an intervention with a ratio of $90,000 per life year gained is considered cost-effective. In the United States there tends to be a general consensus that $50,000 to US$100,000 per life year gained is acceptable,[16] whereas in the United Kingdom, the National Institute for Clinical Effectiveness (NICE) has an implicit threshold of £20,000 to £30,000.[21] In Australia, there is evidence that the Pharmaceutical Benefits Advisory Committee (PBAC) is more likely to recommend the listing of medications with a cost per QALY of less than AUD42,000, and unlikely to recommend a medication for listing where the cost per QALY exceeds AUD76,000 (1998/99 values).[22] Alternative but equivalent ways to present this information are (1) to construct a Cost-Effectiveness Acceptability Curve that shows, over a range of possible thresholds, the probability of being below each threshold; and (2) for each level of the threshold, present the difference between total costs and the product of QALYs gained and the threshold value as the net benefits of treatment.[23] This can be graphed against different values of the threshold with confidence intervals. In the latter case the threshold represents a hypothetical willingness to pay for health gains in terms of QALYs.[23]

The main purpose of cost-effectiveness analysis is to inform decision makers of the most efficient choice in terms of achieving a particular desired outcome (maximum QALYs gained) for least resources. It needs to be recognized that this is not the only objective in health care, and issues of equity and justice may also play a role. For example, one might argue that there is an imperative to act in a setting where a known individual may die if not offered a particular intervention, regardless of cost; this has become known as the "rule of rescue." The rule of rescue is characterized as "the powerful human proclivity to rescue a single identified endangered life, regardless of cost, at the expense of any nameless faces who will therefore be denied health care."[24] This factor may be considered by some to make economic evaluations in the intensive care unit less relevant. That is, it may be perceived that society has a high (or infinite) willingness to pay for any intervention, where the certain alternative is imminent death. Irrespective, economic evaluation has a key role in the critical care setting, at least in decisions such as expanding bed capacity, purchasing a new piece of expensive capital equipment, or including an expensive new treatment in guidelines as a standard of care. In all of these instances, there is an opportunity cost, or benefit foregone within the unit or hospital, if the next best alternative could no longer be offered with available resources.

ANALYTICAL APPROACHES FOR ECONOMIC EVALUATIONS

Numerous methods are available to analysts to compare the costs and effects of alternative interventions. These include trial-based methods and modeled methods.

Trial-Based Economic Evaluations

Trial-based methods involve the economic evaluation being conducted alongside a clinical trial of an intervention. In this case, the case report form (CRF) is expanded from simply collecting health-related information to including health resource utilization (for costing) and an outcome measure appropriate for use in economic evaluation (such as a long-term mortality or a multi-attribute utility instrument for utility calculation) where this was not part of the clinical data collection. Trial-based economic evaluations should be integrated alongside the trial development early to ensure adequate data can be feasibly collected, and that appropriate follow-up can be organized. The advantage of trial-based economic evaluations is that both cost and outcome data come from one group of patients, avoiding the need to incorporate data from many different sources that may be inconsistent.[25] The ideal trial-based economic evaluation is conducted in naturalistic settings, uses a commonly used cost-effective therapy as a comparator, studies the intervention as it would be used in usual care, and has an adequate length of follow-up to assess the full impact of the intervention.[25] Where a trial includes only very specific patients, optimizes treatment with the intervention, and carefully controls other aspects of care, the results may not be generalizable to broader clinical practice, and may not address all of the considerations that go into the decision to adopt a new intervention.[25]

In conducting an economic evaluation alongside a clinical trial, some consideration should be given to power calculations for the economic evaluation to ensure that there are adequate patient numbers to assess the homogeneity of the economic results in a wide range of settings.[25] However, patient numbers in clinical trials are typically based on appropriate powering for the primary clinical endpoint. This is because there is generally a high degree of variability in costing information, leading to impractically large patient numbers required to power an economic study in the traditional sense.

To date, trial-based economic evaluations of critical care interventions are rare. Recently, Peek and colleagues conducted an economic evaluation alongside a randomized controlled trial of extracorporeal membrane oxygenation (ECMO) compared to conventional ventilatory support in patients with severe adult respiratory failure (CESAR).[26] They randomized 180 patients to receive either ECMO or conventional ventilatory management and followed them for 6 months. At 6 months, they found a cost per extra survivor without severe disability of £250,162 (US$404,268), and a cost per QALY of £1,631,124 (US$2,635,933), although they found that the costs were highly variable between patients and the cost-effectiveness ratios showed considerable uncertainty with wide confidence intervals.[26] A lifetime ratio was also calculated using a decision model (see later) based on CESAR trial results and including additional data for predicted lifetime QALYs and health care costs. This found a predicted lifetime incremental cost per QALY (discount rate 3.5%) of £19,252 (US$31,112).[26]

Modeled Economic Evaluations

Modeled methods for economic evaluation involve the synthesis of multiple data sources to construct an economic evaluation. They are commonly undertaken to link additional information to clinical trial data that did not include an economic evaluation, which may include costing data or outcome data such as utility scores. Other reasons for modeling may include, but are not limited to, extrapolation of results beyond the timeframe of a clinical trial or adjustment of some underlying demographic risk parameters to more closely match the trial population to the one of interest.

Modeled economic evaluations usually adopt a decision analytic framework using a treelike structure (a decision tree) or Markov models. Decision trees graphically depict all alternatives for a problem and also stipulate all possible sequelae for each of these alternatives, along with their related probabilities of occurrence and their associated outcomes.[27] They provide an efficient way to capture large volumes of information such as the probability of various events occurring (eg, treatment success, occurrence of side effects), costs of each event, and final outcomes (eg, mortality, life years, or QALYs). When fully populated, decisions trees provide a thorough picture of costs and consequences for all considered treatment alternatives. Each branch of the decision tree can be compared to others to determine incremental costs and benefits to calculate the cost-effectiveness ratio.

An example of a basic decision tree is shown in **Fig. 2**. In this decision tree, the simple comparison of EGDT compared to standard care incorporates the probability of being transferred to the ICU or the ward, with the potential final outcomes of survival or death. The combination of these potential events results in eight discrete "end states," each of which has an associated cost and health outcome that can be compared. Summing the total costs and outcomes for treatment compared to standard care provides the necessary inputs to calculate a cost-effectiveness ratio.

Huang and colleagues conducted a decision analysis of EGDT for severe sepsis and septic shock to explore the potential costs and consequences of EGDT implementation.[28] The decision tree incorporated whether EGDT was delivered by an emergency department (ED)-based team, a mobile team, or an ICU-based team, and final outcomes of survival or death. The estimates of effectiveness and resource use were based on data from the original RCT of EGDT[29] and published sources, and the implementation costs and lifetime projections were modeled from published sources and tested in sensitivity analyses.[28] They found that EGDT implementation had a 99.4% to 99.8% probability of being dominant (saved lives and costs) from the hospital perspective and cost from $2749 (ICU-based) to $7019 (ED-based) per QALY with a 96.7% to 97.7% probability of being less than $20,000 per QALY from the societal perspective.[28]

Similar to decision trees, Markov models (also known as Markov processes) are a common way to structure an analytic problem where there are multiple potential "health states." Whereas decision trees may reflect a chronological ordering of health states or outcomes, Markov models allow the flexibility of movement between health states. Markov models are useful when a decision problem involves risk that is continuous over time, when the timing of events is important, and when important

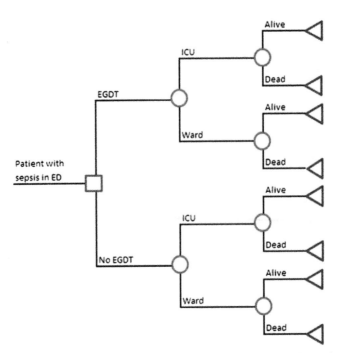

Fig. 2. Graphical representation of a decision tree comparing EGDT and standard care for patients presenting to the ED with severe sepsis. The square node represents a decision node where one must make a choice to implement EGDT or standard care. The circular nodes are chance nodes and represent points at which all events will be determined by chance occurrence and hence are associated with specific probabilities. The triangular nodes are terminal nodes and represent the cumulative costs and effects of each pathway.

events may happen more than once (such as admission to an ICU).[30] Markov models require development of a series of states that must be mutually exclusive (a patient can be in only one state at a time) and collectively exhaustive (the patient has to be in one of the states at all times).[31] Patients move through the model according to probabilities that determine how likely it is to transition from one state to another over a specified period of time (the Markov cycle). Each health state is associated with a certain cost and health outcome for each cycle. To run the Markov model, individual patient cohorts cycle through the different states of the model based on the transition probabilities.[31] The model is run either for a fixed number of cycles or until all patients have entered an absorbing state (a state that they will remain in for all future cycles).[31]

A simple characterization of a Markov model is shown in **Fig. 3**. Patients presenting to the ED with severe sepsis enter the model and receive EGDT or standard care. They are then able to transition into one of three states: they improve and are transferred to the ward, they deteriorate (or do not improve) and are transferred to the intensive care unit, or they die. Patients in the ward can remain on the ward or transition to one of three states: they deteriorate and are admitted to ICU, they improve and are discharged from hospital, or they die. Patients in intensive care can remain in ICU or transition to one of two states: they improve and are transferred to the ward or they die. Patients who have been discharged may transition to death. Transition probabilities are obtained from published data or from expert opinion where published data are not available.

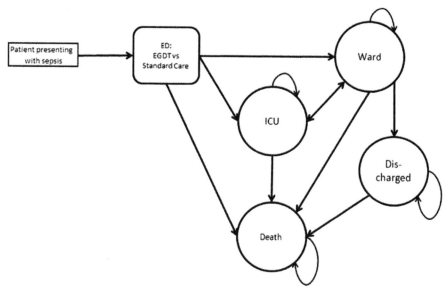

Fig. 3. Graphical representation of a Markov model comparing EGDT and standard care for patients presenting to the ED with severe sepsis. Each circle represents a different health state; arrows indicate the direction of transition from one state to the next.

DEALING WITH UNCERTAINTY

There is inherent uncertainty in the results of economic evaluations because there will never be complete information on all the possible costs and consequences of a particular intervention in a given population.[32] Such uncertainty may be related to the structure of the model or parameter uncertainty related to sampling in the underlying studies of costs and outcomes of treatment. This uncertainty needs to be presented and explored so that informed decisions can be made about whether to adopt a given intervention.

Structural uncertainty relates to the extent to which structural features of the model adequately capture the relevant characteristics of the patient group and intervention being investigated.[32] An example of structural uncertainty is deciding which states to include in a Markov model. Methodological uncertainty relates to evaluation decisions such as the perspective, the discounting procedure and rate, the time horizon, or the source of values for health state preferences. Methodological uncertainty is usually dealt with by prescribing a "reference case" or list of methodological choices to allow comparability between evaluations.[32] Parameter uncertainty relates to the uncertainty about cost and outcome parameters used in the model, with regard to their true value, for example, the unit costs applied to given resources or the mortality rate. Often the base case for the economic evaluation uses a point estimate (such as the point estimate of mortality from an RCT), and the sensitivity analysis varies this value throughout a plausible range (which is often the 95% confidence interval for the point estimate). The uncertain variables in a model can be varied individually (one-way sensitivity analysis) or simultaneously (multiway sensitivity analysis). In addition, some analysts include sampling uncertainty in the model itself by allowing the probability of transition from one health state to another (eg, ICU to death) to be drawn at random from a probability distribution that might describe the underlying mortality data in a meta-analysis of trials. This so called probabilistic sensitivity analysis allows the analyst to put confidence intervals around the point estimate of the incremental cost-effectiveness ratio or net benefit of treatment.

USING THE RESULTS OF AN ECONOMIC EVALUATION

The objective of economic evaluations is to improve decisions about how to allocate health care resources.[7] In assessing the usefulness of the results of an economic evaluation, as with establishing the usefulness of the results of a clinical trial, readers need to establish whether the evaluation methods are appropriate and the results are valid ("Can I believe the results?"). They also need to establish whether the results are generalizable to their clinical practice ("How can I use this with my patients?"). Numerous checklists and critical evaluation guides exist to help readers interpret economic evaluations.[7,8]

Following on from the consideration of trial-based and modeled economic evaluations, one may consider that trial-based methods, where conducted appropriately, have a high degree of validity due to their homogeneous patient population and consistent application of an intervention. Modeled evaluations may be more difficult to interpret for validity where they combine data from multiple sources and the quality of these underlying inputs are not provided or adequately assessed. However, modeling may be a legitimate and appropriate way in which to apply the results of a trial-based evaluation to a different setting, for example, via extrapolation of results, adjustment of baseline risk levels, or focused subgroup analysis.

In assessing validity, readers must consider all of the aspects of economic evaluations described in this article, such as what alternatives were chosen, how costs were measured, whether all relevant costs were identified, how outcomes were determined, how discounting was performed, what uncertainty exists, and how sensitivity analyses were performed. In assessing generalizability, readers need to consider whether, for example, the resource use is similar to the resources used in their clinical practices. For example, in Australia, ICU patients are nursed with a 1:1 ratio, whereas patients are nursed with higher ratios in some other countries. In an intervention that affects length of stay, the costs will differ depending on the nursing ratio, which will affect the resulting cost-effectiveness ratio. Reasons why data in an economic evaluation may not be generalizable to a reader's practice include difference in the availability of alternative treatments, in clinical practice patterns, or in relative prices.[7]

SUMMARY

Resources in the health care system are limited, and with an increasing demand for health care services, economic evaluations are becoming increasingly important. Given the high cost of many critical care interventions and the increasing demand for critical care services, it is imperative that new interventions are assessed not only for their efficacy, but for their cost-effectiveness. Economic evaluations of critical care interventions are becoming increasingly common and it is essential that clinicians understand the concepts and methods of economic evaluation so that they can appreciate the rationale behind decisions that need to be made about the best use of limited resources and are able to use that information to inform those decisions.

REFERENCES

1. Pines JM, Fager SS, Milzman DP. A review of costing methodologies in critical care studies. J Crit Care 2002;17(3):181–6.

2. Heyland DK, Kernerman P, Gafni A, et al. Economic evaluations in the critical care literature: do they help us improve the efficiency of our unit? Crit Care Med 1996;24(9): 1591–8.

3. Gyldmark M. A review of cost studies of intensive care units: problems with the cost concept. Crit Care Med 1995;23(5):964–72.

4. Cox HL, Laupland KB, Manns BJ. Economic evaluation in critical care medicine. J Crit Care 2006;21(2):117–24.

5. American Thoracic Society. Understanding Costs and Cost-Effectiveness in Critical Care: Report from the Second American Thoracic Society Workshop in Outcomes Research. Am J Respir Crit Care Med 2002;165:540–50.

6. Chalfin DB, Cohen IL, Lambrinos J. The economics and cost-effectiveness of critical care medicine. Intensive Care Med 1995;21(11):952–61.

7. Drummond MF, O'Brien B, Stoddart GL, et al. Methods for the economic evaluation of health care programs. 2nd edition. New York: Oxford University Press; 1997.

8. Drummond MF, Jefferson TO. Guidelines for authors and peer reviewers of economic submissions to the BMJ. The BMJ Economic Evaluation Working Party. BMJ 1996; 313(7052):275–83.

9. Angus DC, Carlet J. Surviving intensive care: a report from the 2002 Brussels Roundtable. Intensive Care Med 2003;29(3):368–77.

10. EuroQol—a new facility for the measurement of health-related quality of life. The EuroQol Group. Health Policy 1990;16(3):199–208.

11. Brazier J, Roberts J, Deverill M. The estimation of a preference-based measure of health from the SF-36. J Health Econ 2002;21(2):271–92.

12. Sintonen H. The 15D instrument of health-related quality of life: properties and applications. Ann Med 2001;33(5):328–36.

13. Feeny D, Furlong W, Torrance GW, et al. Multiattribute and single-attribute utility functions for the health utilities index mark 3 system. Med Care 2002;40(2): 113–28.

14. Hawthorne G, Richardson J, Day N, et al. Construction and utility scaling of the Assessment of Quality of Life (AQoL) instrument: Centre for Health Program Evaluation, Monash University; 2000. Working paper 101.

15. Weinstein MC, Siegel JE, Gold MR, et al. Recommendations of the Panel on Cost-Effectiveness in Health and Medicine. JAMA 1996;276(15):1253–8.

16. Talmor D, Shapiro N, Greenberg D, et al. When is critical care medicine cost-effective? A systematic review of the cost-effectiveness literature. Crit Care Med 2006;34(11): 2738–47.

17. Pandharipande PP, Pun BT, Herr DL, et al. Effect of sedation with dexmedetomidine vs lorazepam on acute brain dysfunction in mechanically ventilated patients: the MENDS randomized controlled trial. JAMA 2007;298(22):2644–53.

18. Coughlin M, Angus D. Assessing cost effectiveness in the intensive care unit. In: Hall J, Schmidt G, Wood L, editors. Principles of critical care. 3rd edition. New York: McGraw-Hill; 2005. Available at: http://www.accessmedicine.com. Accessed June 8, 2009.

19. Quartin AA, Schein RM, Kett DH, et al. Magnitude and duration of the effect of sepsis on survival. Department of Veterans Affairs Systemic Sepsis Cooperative Studies Group. JAMA 1997;277(13):1058–63.

20. Timmers TK, Verhofstad MH, Moons KG, et al. Long-term quality of life after surgical intensive care admission. Arch Surg 2011;146(4):412–8.

21. McCabe C, Claxton K, Culyer AJ. The NICE cost-effectiveness threshold: what it is and what that means. Pharmacoeconomics 2008;26(9):733–44.

22. George B, Harris A, Mitchell A. Cost-effectiveness analysis and the consistency of decision making: evidence from pharmaceutical reimbursement in Australia (1991 to 1996). Pharmacoeconomics 2001;19(11):1103–9.

23. Willan A, Briggs A. Statistical analysis of cost-effectiveness data. West Sussex (UK): John Wiley & Sons; 2006.

24. Osborne M, Evans TW. Allocation of resources in intensive care: a transatlantic perspective. Lancet 1994;343(8900):778–80.

25. Glick HA, Doshi JA, Sonnard SS, et al. Economic evaluation in clinical trials. New York: Oxford University Press; 2007.

26. Peek GJ, Mugford M, Tiruvoipati R, et al. Efficacy and economic assessment of conventional ventilatory support versus extracorporeal membrane oxygenation for severe adult respiratory failure (CESAR): a multicentre randomised controlled trial. Lancet 2009;374(9698):1351–63.

27. Chalfin DB. Decision analysis in critical care medicine. Crit Care Clin 1999;15(3):647–61, viii.

28. Huang DT, Clermont G, Dremsizov TT, et al. Implementation of early goal-directed therapy for severe sepsis and septic shock: a decision analysis. Crit Care Med 2007;35(9):2090–100.

29. Rivers E, Nguyen B, Havstad S, et al. Early goal-directed therapy in the treatment of severe sepsis and septic shock. N Engl J Med 2001;345(19):1368–77.

30. Sonnenberg FA, Beck JR. Markov models in medical decision making: a practical guide. Med Decis Making 1993;13(4):322–38.

31. Kreke JE, Schaefer AJ, Roberts MS. Simulation and critical care modeling. Curr Opin Crit Care 2004;10(5):395–8.

32. Bilcke J, Beutels P, Brisson M, et al. Accounting for methodological, structural, and parameter uncertainty in decision-analytic models: a practical guide. Med Decis Making 2011;31(4):675–92.

Economics of ICU Organization and Management

Hannah Wunsch, MD, MSc[a,b,]*, Hayley Gershengorn, MD[c],
Damon C. Scales, MD, PhD[d,]

KEYWORDS

- Critical care • Intensive care unit • Length of stay • Staffing
- Organization • Economics

Intensive care is an integral but expensive component of healthcare in developed countries.[1] An estimate in the United States is that fully 2% of the population receives intensive care every year,[2] and overall the percentage of patients who receive intensive care before they die is increasing.[3,4] Projections of the need for mechanical ventilation predict an exponential growth in the coming years due to the aging population and their over-representation among mechanically ventilated cohorts[5]; this increase in need for mechanical ventilation will be associated with increasing costs of intensive care.[6,7] Much of the focus of intensive care is on improvements in technology for organ support and resuscitation. Yet quality healthcare also involves appropriate organization of resources, with the potential to both impact patient outcomes and the costs of the care provided. These economic considerations are likely to become increasingly important as the demand for critical care increases in the face of limited resources.

The economics of organizing the delivery of intensive care can focus on the management of human resources and operating costs within an ICU itself, or the use

Funding was provided by award K08AG038477 from the National Institute on Aging to Hannah Wunsch.

The authors have nothing to disclose.

[a] Department of Anesthesiology, Columbia University, 622 West 168th Street, New York, NY 10032, USA

[b] Department of Epidemiology, Mailman School of Public Health, 722 West 168th Street, Columbia University, New York, NY 10032, USA

[c] Division of Pulmonary, Critical Care, and Sleep Medicine, Beth Israel Medical Center, First Avenue at 16th Street, 7 Dazian, New York, NY 10003, USA

[d] Interdepartmental Division of Critical Care Medicine, Department of Critical Care, University of Toronto, Sunnybrook Health Sciences Centre, 2075 Bayview Avenue, Room D108, Toronto, ON M4N 3M5, Canada

* Corresponding author.

E-mail address: hw2125@columbia.edu

of ICU resources within a healthcare system. This article will focus on both these perspectives, emphasizing issues related to optimal staffing and the economic consequences of different staffing choices.

PERSPECTIVE REGARDING COSTS

The costs of providing critical care can be considered in short-term and long-term time horizons and are incurred to varying degrees by patients, hospitals, insurance companies, the government or other payer, and society as a whole. Thus, the first question to ask when evaluating the economic impact of any organizational change affecting the ICU is which party actually accrues a cost change.[8] In this article, we will primarily focus on the potential economic implications of organization and management choices from the perspective of the individual hospital.

Fixed Versus Variable Costs In the ICU

Hospital costs are composed of fixed and variable costs. In brief, the *fixed costs* remain constant and are independent of small changes in the number of patients being cared for in the hospital. They also generally reflect the operational costs required to provide care.[9] Examples of fixed costs in the ICU include staff salaries, the money paid to purchase mechanical ventilators, and the maintenance required on the building. *Variable costs* are the hospital costs associated with the care of individual patients, and will fluctuate with patient volumes. Examples of variable costs are the costs of specific medications the patient receives or the cost of an additional central venous catheter inserted.[10] The majority of costs associated with care in the hospital are fixed costs, often estimated to account for over 80% of total costs.[9] Whether or not hospital (or ICU) beds are occupied, the hospital continues to pay the fixed costs of care, and therefore most cost reductions associated with any system change will be small if due to changes in variable costs only.

The economics of intensive care from the perspective of the hospital also depend on how a hospital is reimbursed by a health system.[8] For example, under one type of payment system, a hospital receives a set amount of money for the care of all patients, regardless of the number that are actually admitted. Another option is a fixed level of reimbursement to the hospital to provide care for each patient admitted with a specific diagnosis or surgical procedure. In these situations, the actual components of treatment that are provided to an individual patient are not reimbursed separately, but instead the hospital receives a lump sum based upon expected costs. In a "per diem" model, the hospital is paid an additional sum for each day that a patient remains hospitalized. Hospitals can also be paid using a fee-for-service model, receiving a sum of money for each additional test, procedure, medication, etc that is provided to each patient. Within each of these payment schemes, there are opportunities for the hospital to change the system to maximize revenue. In this article, we primarily consider the actual costs of providing treatment when discussing strategies for reducing total costs, rather than strategies to improve the economic outlook for the hospital based on different payment schemes.

COSTS WITHIN THE ICU
Decreasing Length of Stay

Many studies in critical care target reductions in ICU length of stay and equate this outcome with a "cost savings." In reality, large cost savings will only be realized if the reductions in ICU length of stay result in a reduced number of total admissions and consequent reductions in number of ICU beds and fixed costs of care.[11] In addition, one must be cognizant of the concept of "cost-shifting," in which reductions in costs in one area are accompanied by increases in costs elsewhere in order to address clinical needs. In most situations the actual cost savings associated with decreased ICU length of stay therefore comprise only a small fraction of total costs. For example, Kahn and colleagues analyzed the potential cost savings attributable to reductions in ICU length of stay for ICU survivors who had received mechanical ventilation and ICU admission of more than 3 days. The authors found that the mean variable costs of the last day in the ICU was $397, while the cost of the next day on the hospital ward was $279; thus, reducing ICU length of stay by 1 day would only result in a cost savings of 0.2% of all hospital expenditure for that patient.[12] Conversely, if there is typically high demand for ICU resources (and the absolute number of patients in the ICU remains relatively constant), reducing ICU length of stay can paradoxically increase variable costs because higher acuity patients requiring more intensive and expensive treatments replace the lower-acuity patients who are discharged.[12] Moreover, the overall economic effect of accommodating an additional ICU patient may be different depending on the type of ICU and the type of patient. For example, if any decrease in one patient's ICU length of stay helps avoid the cancellation of an elective surgery such as coronary artery bypass grafting for another patient, the actual economic impact on the hospital may be different than providing admission for an additional patient with pneumonia, but will also depend on how the hospital is reimbursed, as described earlier. In this article we address specific organizational aspects of the ICU by focusing on the actual costs incurred by providing direct care and, where possible, avoid inferences based on economic implications of reducing ICU length of stay. However, we generally consider interventions that decrease ICU length of stay to be desirable.

Staffing

The largest and primarily fixed costs of operating an ICU are staff salaries, which are estimated to account for over 50% of fixed costs for all hospitalized patients in the United States[9] and 33% to 69% of total ICU costs in other countries (**Fig. 1**).[13–20]

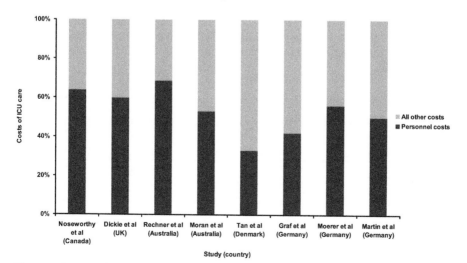

Fig. 1. Estimates of personnel costs associated with the ICU.

Staffing patterns in the ICU vary markedly between ICUs and between health systems, with variations in the specialty of the physicians, nurse-to-patient ratios, and the presence of other healthcare professionals on the team. Yet, the large proportion of costs in the ICU taken up by the compensation for its staff seems to be relatively consistent across many countries, despite the different staffing patterns and health-care systems.

Nursing

Nurses are an integral, if not the most vital, component of all ICU teams, but perhaps paradoxically, nurse-to-patient staffing ratios and other issues related to the provision of ICU nursing care differ from country to country, from region to region, and even may differ between ICUs in a particular hospital. One European study, for example, from the 1990s found that the majority of ICU nurses cared for 2 patients but also observed substantial variation between the planned nurse-to-patient ratios and actual staffing ratios in the ICU.[21] Studies conducted outside of the ICU have shown that higher nurse-to-patient ratios and more highly trained nursing staff are associated with fewer adverse events[22] and possibly decreased hospital mortality.[23] Fewer data are available to inform the most cost-effective nurse-to-patient ratio in an ICU, although some studies have suggested that higher nursing ratios decrease adverse event rates and lead to better patient outcomes.[22,24,25] Obviously, maintaining a higher nurse-to-patient ratio increases the fixed costs of intensive care and is a major barrier to providing one-on-one nursing in many ICUs (**Table 1**). It is also possible that savings associated with reductions in adverse events for patients could offset the higher fixed costs of higher nursing ratios, but this possibility remains speculative. Some ICUs have adopted a "flex" system that flexibly schedules nurses based on the anticipated workload in the unit at that time, rather than staffing based on the number of admitted patients or total beds. This structure may be financially beneficial for the hospital and may also improve nursing satisfaction by matching staff to workload demands.[26] However, this model may also result in unpredictable working hours and salaries for individual nurses.

Intensivist staffing

A great deal of attention is focused on the role of intensivists in the management of critically ill patients, particularly in the United States where there is a mix of staffing systems with only approximately one-third of ICUs covered by intensivists.[27] Overall, most studies demonstrate that intensivist staffing in the ICU improves clinical

Table 1
Examples of potential effects on hospital costs of different changes to ICU organiz±ation and management

Organizational Change	Possible Clinical Outcome	Fixed Costs	Variable Costs
Closing ICU beds	Unclear	Decreased	Decreased
Intensivist staffing	Decreased mortality	Increased	Unclear
Pharmacist staffing	Fewer adverse drug events, deceased LOS	Increased	Decreased
Lower nurse to patient ratio	Fewer adverse events, decreased LOS	Increased	Unclear
Checklist prompter	Decreased mortality, decreased LOS	Increased	Decreased

outcomes[28] and both the American College of Critical Care and the Society of Critical Care Medicine recommend intensivist coverage.[29] However, these studies have varied in the definition of a "closed" or "open" ICU and the number of hours of intensivist coverage and are hampered by potential selection biases associated with which patients received intensivist coverage as well as other factors such as the type of ICU, concomitant staffing patterns, and ICU culture.[30,31] Few studies have considered the cost-effectiveness of intensivist staffing. One simulation of intensivist implementation demonstrated cost savings (for the hospital), depending on the size of the ICU, but involved many large assumptions to draw conclusions regarding the impact of intensivists on the hospital system as a whole.[32]

Recent discussions have questioned whether 24-hour in-house intensivist coverage might lead to additional improvements in patient outcomes compared to daytime-only intensivist coverage.[33] One study demonstrated improved compliance with recommended processes of care, but no effect on hospital mortality with 24-hour in-house coverage.[34] Recent work by Banerjee and colleagues examined 24-hour in-house intensivist coverage (vs daytime only) and demonstrated a decreased length of stay for the sickest patients admitted at night and cost savings associated with the decreased length of stay.[35] The study did include estimates of the costs of additional intensivists, but did not clearly differentiate between fixed and marginal costs of care, thus potentially overestimating the cost savings associated with the decreased length of stay.

Multidisciplinary teams

Nonphysician team members have a large role in the ICU.[36,37] Data suggest that multidisciplinary teams on rounds can potentially impact the mortality[38] and length of stay of patients in the ICU.[39] However, expanding the membership of the multidisciplinary team, especially non-nursing healthcare workers, may also increase fixed costs in an ICU (**Table 1**).

Pharmacists have become an integral component of many ICU teams and several studies demonstrate the economic impact of clinical pharmacists in the ICU. One study in particular detailed the changes made in medication management with the input of a clinical pharmacist over a 3-month period, with a substantial portion of the consultations (47.1%) resulting in decreased drug costs.[40] More recent studies examined the impact of clinical pharmacists on management of particular groups of patients, such as critically ill patients with thromboembolic or infarction-related events[41] and infections.[42] Both studies demonstrated that direct involvement of pharmacists in care led to decreased charges for medications. However, it is important to note that the decreased variable costs may be offset by the fixed costs of the additional salaries.

Perhaps the more important benefit of pharmacists is the potential to decrease adverse drug events.[43] Preventable adverse drug events in the ICU may occur twice as frequently as on the regular hospital ward, primarily due to the greater number of drugs ordered in the ICU,[44] thus making the ICU a prime target for improvement in this area. One study demonstrated a decrease in prescribing errors by two-thirds with the addition of a senior pharmacist on rounds in the ICU.[45] The cost-effectiveness of pharmacists should therefore consider not only the pharmacist's salary and prescribing costs but also the potential reduction in the incidence of expensive complications.

Respiratory therapists are common in North American ICUs and often assume important clinical roles, especially with respect to ventilator management. The use of respiratory therapists varies in other countries. Outside of the ICU, respiratory therapist–initiated treatment protocols have led to better compliance with institutional algorithms for care.[46,47] In the ICU, respiratory therapists have been shown to improve compliance with weaning protocols and decreased duration of mechanical ventilation.[48,49] Guidelines for weaning and discontinuing ventilatory support recommend that protocols designed for nonphysician health-care professionals should be developed and implemented by ICUs.[50] However, the impact of respiratory therapists on both patient mortality[51] and the economics of care is still not well defined.

The role of the physical therapist in the ICU appears to be evolving to include early rehabilitation, including mobilization of mechanically ventilated patients. Several recent studies have suggested that early rehabilitation may lead to improved patient outcomes, including functional status[52,53] and length of stay.[52–54] The full economic impact along with the cost-effectiveness of this intervention requires further study, but limited evidence suggests that this therapy may not lead to increased costs of care, even after accounting for the salaries of the physical therapy team.[52] Further research to evaluate the impact of this intervention is required, but the potential for large systemwide savings may also exist if some of these patients no longer require additional care in nursing or rehabilitation facilities due to early intervention.

Finally, the role of a palliative care team in the ICU, either as a separate consult team or as part of the ICU team itself, is still being defined, and the potential financial implications are not yet well explored. No studies have specifically addressed the financial impact of palliative care in patients in the ICU, but introducing these teams may lead to less use of intensive care (in subsets of patients)[55] and reductions in ICU length of stay.[56,57] However, the cost savings of these interventions may be limited since these patients represent a relatively small proportion of patients who (may) be cared for in the ICU and are likely to influence only the marginal costs of care.[11] It remains unknown whether reducing use of ICU at the end of life through aggressive palliative care can lead to any substantial impact on costs of care.

Standardization of Care

Health technology in the ICU, such as mechanical ventilators, pulmonary artery catheters, and other monitoring devices, may represent either fixed or variable costs. Many of these ICU technologies have a limited evidence base supporting their use and could be considered targets for cost-reduction strategies. The use of intensive care technology has been shown to vary widely among different intensivists working in the same ICU, with no discernible variation in patient outcomes. In one study, the daily discretionary costs of care varied by 43% across different intensivists, with a mean difference of $1,003 per admission and no differences in ICU length of stay or hospital mortality.[58] Reducing use of technology and equipment that have not been linked to improved patient outcomes will likely decrease costs[59] but can be slow to occur if clinicians consider these to be an integral part of ICU care. A recent example of changing practice is the use of pulmonary artery catheters; after multiple studies failed to demonstrate any clinical benefit associated with their systematic use in different ICU populations, the frequency of insertion has dropped dramatically in the United States.[60,61]

Standardization of treatment approaches and the use of protocols to help organize ICU care can help reduce the use of unproven and expensive treatments (or at least ensure that they are used only in situations that are supported by strong levels of evidence) and also may lead to increased use of evidence-based therapies and improved patient outcomes. There are many ways to approach standardization of care, which include the addition of multidisciplinary staff (as described earlier), the implementation of checklists,[62,63] prompting and the use of clinical reminders,[63] and the adoption of clinical protocols and treatment "bundles."[64] Some of these options have been examined as individual components (such as checklists[65]) and others as "bundles" of care to be delivered together.[64,66] The combination of checklists on rounds with a "prompter" to ensure that the elements of the checklist were addressed was associated in one single-center study with decreases in mortality and length of ICU stay, potentially decreasing variable costs associated with care.[63] However, the fixed costs of requiring additional staff to act as "prompter" may offset the potential economic benefit of this intervention (see **Table 1**).

Many ICUs and hospitals have implemented protocols to limit the use of expensive technologies and treatments to their appropriate and evidence-based indications as a strategy to reduce costs and "indication creep." For example, there has been a substantial increase in off-label use of recombinant factor VIIa,[67] with little evidence to support its administration in many cases.[68] In the ICU, even a test as basic as an arterial blood gas may be subject to overuse, with one study demonstrating a substantial decrease in the number of arterial blood gas requests with implementation of guidelines and feedback.[69]

COSTS WITHIN THE HEALTHCARE SYSTEM
Organization of Admission and Discharge Practices and Alternatives to Care

Since ICU care is almost always more expensive than the care provided on a general ward,[12] choosing to *not* admit a patient to the ICU will likely decrease the costs of care for that individual. However, such decisions will also likely lead to worse outcomes if appropriate and potentially life-saving treatments are withheld; decreasing the use of intensive care is therefore only a feasible approach to decreasing costs if the admission to the ICU is not appropriate. One study examined the factors associated with being a "high-performance" ICU (defined as having a standardized mortality ratio of 1.0 or less) and found that these high-performing units all had ICU directors (or a designee) who were authorized to refuse admission to patients not meeting appropriate criteria and to triage requested admissions to extended-stay recovery rooms and intermediate care areas.[70] Cost savings for the hospital may also be realized if subacutely or chronically critically ill patients are discharged more expeditiously from the ICU, although as noted earlier, decreasing ICU length of stay by small amounts (such as a single day) may do little to impact costs of care.[12] However, patients with ongoing respiratory failure traditionally have had few options for care once their needs for acute intensive care are over, yet often stay in an ICU for extended periods. Different institutions attempt to accommodate these patients outside the traditional ICU setting in different manners. The designation of a flexibly sized section of the surgical ICU for the "subacutely ill" allowed for reductions in costly resources (eg, nursing) without the additional cost of building a separate step-down facility.[71] Similarly, several studies demonstrate that the creation of a physically separate step-down unit may result in reduced costs of care.[72–75] Another option in some hospitals, particularly in the United States, is to transfer patients quickly out of the acute hospital to receive prolonged care elsewhere. The use of long-term acute care facilities (which can care for mechanically ventilated patients) in the United States has increased dramatically over the past decade.[76] Whether the movement of patients to these facilities is cost effective for the healthcare system as a whole is unclear, but there may be a substantial decrease in costs for the acute care hospital if patients are discharged much earlier.

Regionalization

A broader approach to triage of patients to the most appropriate setting is regionalization of ICU beds and care of ICU patients, particularly mechanically ventilated patients. In the United States this idea has been proposed based on data suggesting that outcomes may be improved for mechanically ventilated patients cared for at higher-volume hospitals.[77] Regionalized systems exist for both trauma and neonatal care,[78,79] and some regionalization occurs in most countries, either through formal systems[80] or informal networks.[81] However, the barriers to complete regionalization of intensive care are substantial, including concerns regarding strain on patients' families, lack of strong central authority to organize triage, and the potential to overwhelm capacity at larger hospitals.[82] The impact of regionalization of intensive care for the economics of hospitals is also uncertain, with concern that smaller hospitals may be hurt financially, while larger hospitals receiving patients may not have enough resources.[83]

Alternatively, telemedicine could allow for an increased reach of critical care expertise in remote ICUs by providing access to intensivists. These physicians may offer either monitoring or consultation as needed, and theoretically provide the associated benefits for patient care seen in studies of intensivist staffing.[28] However, the results are inconsistent[84]; two multicenter studies were unable to demonstrate an association between the use of telemedicine and patient outcomes,[85,86] while one has shown improvements for patients,[87] and another demonstrated some economic benefit.[88]

Assessing the potential impact of telemedicine programs is hampered by the fact that their adoption has often been studied in ICUs that already have high staffing ratios. The true benefit may be found only in small hospitals with limited access to intensivist care. Telemedicine could also be used as a tool to improve the implementation of specific interventions, and to facilitate adherence to current best practice, such as lung protective ventilation or early-goal directed therapy.[89]

SUMMARY

The ICU is a complex system and the economic implications of altering care patterns in the ICU can be difficult to unravel. While the clinical impact of many aspects of organization and management have been studied in the ICU, few studies have specifically examined the economics of implementing organizational and management changes. Even fewer have acknowledged the many competing economic interests of patient, hospital, payer, and society. It does appear, however, that for certain aspects of ICU organization (eg, the inclusion of a staff pharmacist on a multidisciplinary ICU team), there may be an alignment of clinical and financial goals for all parties. With continuously increasing healthcare costs there is a great need for more studies focused on economics to inform the optimal organization of the ICU. Ideally these studies should not focus solely on reductions in ICU length of stay but should strive to measure the true costs of care within a given healthcare system.

REFERENCES

1. Wunsch H, Angus DC, Harrison DA, et al. Variation in critical care services across North America and Western Europe. Crit Care Med 2008;36:2787–9.
2. Kersten A, Milbrandt EB, Rahim MT, et al. How big is critical care in the U.S.? [abstract]. Crit Care Med 2003;31(Suppl):A8.
3. Barnato AE, McClellan MB, Kagay CR, et al. Trends in inpatient treatment intensity among Medicare beneficiaries at the end of life. Health Serv Res 2004;39:363–75.
4. Angus DC, Barnato AE, Linde-Zwirble WT, et al. Use of intensive care at the end of life in the United States: an epidemiologic study. Crit Care Med 2004;32:638–43.
5. Carson SS, Cox CE, Holmes GM, et al. The changing epidemiology of mechanical ventilation: a population-based study. J Intensive Care Med 2006;21:173–82.

6. Fisher ES, Bynum JP, Skinner JS. Slowing the growth of health care costs–lessons from regional variation. N Engl J Med 2009;360:849–52.
7. Sutherland JM, Fisher ES, Skinner JS. Getting past denial—the high cost of health care in the United States. N Engl J Med 2009;361:1227–30.
8. Kahn JM. Understanding economic outcomes in critical care. Curr Opin Crit Care 2006;12:399–404.
9. Roberts RR, Frutos PW, Ciavarella GG, et al. Distribution of variable vs fixed costs of hospital care. JAMA 1999;281:644–9.
10. Rossi C, Simini B, Brazzi L, et al. Variable costs of ICU patients: a multicenter prospective study. Intensive Care Med 2006;32:545–52.
11. Luce JM, Rubenfeld GD. Can health care costs be reduced by limiting intensive care at the end of life? Am J Respir Crit Care Med 2002;165:750–54.
12. Kahn JM, Rubenfeld GD, Rohrbach J, et al. Cost savings attributable to reductions in intensive care unit length of stay for mechanically ventilated patients. Med Care 2008;46:1226–33.
13. Noseworthy TW, Konopad E, Shustack A, et al. Cost accounting of adult intensive care: methods and human and capital inputs. Crit Care Med 1996;24:1168–72.
14. Dickie H, Vedio A, Dundas R, et al. Relationship between TISS and ICU cost. Intensive Care Med 1998;24:1009–17.
15. Rechner IJ, Lipman J. The costs of caring for patients in a tertiary referral Australian intensive care unit. Anaesth intensive Care 2005;33:477.
16. Moran JL, Peisach AR, Solomon PJ, et al. Cost calculation and prediction in adult intensive care: a ground-up utilization study. Anaesth Intensive Care 2004;32:787–97.
17. Tan SS, Hakkaart-van Roijen L, Al MJ, et al. Review of a large clinical series: a microcosting study of intensive care unit stay in the Netherlands. J Intensive Care Med 2008;23:250–7.
18. Graf J, Graf C, Janssens U. Analysis of resource use and cost-generating factors in a German medical intensive care unit employing the Therapeutic Intervention Scoring System (TISS-28). Intensive Care Med 2002;28:324–31.
19. Moerer O, Plock E, Mgbor U, et al. A German national prevalence study on the cost of intensive care: an evaluation from 51 intensive care units. Crit Care (Lond Engl) 2007;11:R69.
20. Martin J, Neurohr C, Bauer M, et al. Cost of intensive care in a German hospital: cost-unit accounting based on the InEK matrix. Anaesthesist 2008;57:50512.
21. Moreno R, Reis MD. Nursing staff in intensive care in Europe: the mismatch between planning and practice. Chest 1998;113:752–8.
22. Heinz D. Hospital nurse staffing and patient outcomes: a review of current literature. Dimens Crit Care Nursing 2004;23:44.
23. Needleman J, Buerhaus P, Pankratz VS, et al. Nurse staffing and inpatient hospital mortality. N Engl J Med 2011;364:1037–45.
24. Amaravadi RK, Dimick JB, Pronovost PJ, et al. ICU nurse-to-patient ratio is associated with complications and resource use after esophagectomy. Intensive Care Med 2000;26:1857–62.
25. Binnekade JM, Vroom MB, de Mol BA, et al. The quality of intensive care nursing before, during, and after the introduction of nurses without ICU-training. Heart Lung 2003;32:190–6.
26. Cho SH, June KJ, Kim YM, et al. Nurse staffing, quality of nursing care and nurse job outcomes in intensive care units. J Clin Nursing 2009;18:1729–37.

27. Angus DC, Shorr AF, White A, et al. Critical care delivery in the United States: distribution of services and compliance with Leapfrog recommendations. Crit Care Med 2006;34:1016–24.
28. Pronovost PJ, Angus DC, Dorman T, et al. Physician staffing patterns and clinical outcomes in critically ill patients: a systematic review. JAMA 2002;288:2151–62.
29. Haupt MT, Bekes CE, Brilli RJ, et al. Guidelines on critical care services and personnel: Recommendations based on a system of categorization of three levels of care. Crit Care Med 2003;31:2677–83.
30. Levy MM, Rapoport J, Lemeshow S, et al. Association between critical care physician management and patient mortality in the intensive care unit. Ann Intern Med 2008; 148:801–9.
31. Pronovost PJ, Jenckes MW, Dorman T, et al. Organizational characteristics of intensive care units related to outcomes of abdominal aortic surgery. JAMA 1999; 281:1310–7.
32. Pronovost PJ, Needham DM, Waters H, et al. Intensive care unit physician staffing: financial modeling of the Leapfrog standard. Crit Care Med 2006;34(3 Suppl): S18–24.
33. Sapirstein A, Needham D, Pronovost PJ. 24-hour intensivist staffing: Balancing benefits and costs. Crit Care Med 2008;36:367–8.
34. Gajic O, Afessa B, Hanson AC, et al. Effect of 24-hour mandatory versus on-demand critical care specialist presence on quality of care and family and provider satisfaction in the intensive care unit of a teaching hospital. Crit Care Med 2008;36:36–44.
35. Banerjee R, Naessens JM, Seferian EG, et al. Economic implications of nighttime attending intensivist coverage in a medical intensive care unit. Crit Care Med 2011; 39:1257–62.
36. Curtis JR, Cook DJ, Wall RJ, et al. Intensive care unit quality improvement: A "how-to" guide for the interdisciplinary team. Crit Care Med 2006;34:211–8.
37. Nguyen YL, Wunsch H, Angus DC. Critical care: the impact of organization and management on outcomes. Curr Opin Crit Care 2010;16:487–92.
38. Kim MM, Barnato AE, Angus DC, et al. The effect of multidisciplinary care teams on intensive care unit mortality. Arch Intern Med 2010;170:369–76.
39. Smyrnios NA, Connolly A, Wilson MM, et al. Effects of a multifaceted, multidisciplinary, hospital-wide quality improvement program on weaning from mechanical ventilation. Crit Care Med 2002;30:1224–30.
40. Montazeri M, Cook DJ. Impact of a clinical pharmacist in a multidisciplinary intensive care unit. Crit Care Med 1994;22:1044–8.
41. MacLaren R, Bond CA. Effects of pharmacist participation in intensive care units on clinical and economic outcomes of critically ill patients with thromboembolic or infarction-related events. Pharmacotherapy 2009;29:761–8.
42. MacLaren R, Bond CA, Martin SJ, et al. Clinical and economic outcomes of involving pharmacists in the direct care of critically ill patients with infections. Crit Care Med 2008;36:3184–9.
43. Horn E, Jacobi J. The critical care clinical pharmacist: evolution of an essential team member. Crit Care Med 2006;34(3 Suppl):S46–S51.
44. Cullen DJ, Sweitzer BJ, Bates DW, et al. Preventable adverse drug events in hospitalized patients: a comparative study of intensive care and general care units. Crit Care Med 1997;25:1289–97.
45. Leape LL, Cullen DJ, Clapp MD, et al. Pharmacist participation on physician rounds and adverse drug events in the intensive care unit. JAMA 1999;282:267–70.

46. Kollef MH, Shapiro SD, Clinkscale D, et al. The effect of respiratory therapist-initiated treatment protocols on patient outcomes and resource utilization. Chest 2000;117: 467–75.
47. Stoller J, Mascha E, Kester L, et al. Randomized controlled trial of physician-directed versus respiratory therapy consult service-directed respiratory care to adult non-ICU inpatients. Am J Respir Crit Care Med 1998;158:1068–75.
48. Ely E, Bennett P, Bowton D, et al. Large Scale implementation of a respiratory therapist- driven protocol for ventilator weaning. Am J Respir Crit Care Med 1999; 159:439–46.
49. Marelich GP, Murin S, Battistella F, et al. Protocol weaning of mechanical ventilation in medical and surgical patients by respiratory care practitioners and nurses. Chest 2000;118:459.
50. MacIntyre NR, Cook DJ, Ely EW Jr, et al. Evidence-based guidelines for weaning and discontinuing ventilatory support: a collective task force facilitated by the American College of Chest Physicians; the American Association for Respiratory Care; and the American College of Crit Care Med. Chest 2001;120(6 Suppl):375S–95S.
51. Blackwood B, Alderdice F, Burns KEA, et al. Use of weaning protocols for reducing duration of mechanical ventilation in critically ill adult patients: cochrane systematic review and meta-analysis. BMJ (Clin Res Ed) 2011;342:c7237.
52. Morris PE, Goad A, Thompson C, et al. Early intensive care unit mobility therapy in the treatment of acute respiratory failure. Crit Care Med 2008;36:2238–43.
53. Schweickert WD, Pohlman MC, Pohlman AS, et al. Early physical and occupational therapy in mechanically ventilated, critically ill patients: a randomised controlled trial. Lancet 2009;373(9678):1874–82.
54. Needham DM, Korupolu R. Rehabilitation quality improvement in an intensive care unit setting: implementation of a quality improvement model. Top Stroke Rehabil 2010;17:271–81.
55. Morrison RS, Penrod JD, Cassel JB, et al. Cost savings associated with US hospital palliative care consultation programs. Arch Intern Med 2008;168:1783–90.
56. Penrod JD, Deb P, Dellenbaugh C, et al. Hospital-based palliative care consultation: effects on hospital cost. J Palliat Med 2010;13:973–9.
57. Norton SA, Hogan LA, Holloway RG, et al. Proactive palliative care in the medical intensive care unit: effects on length of stay for selected high-risk patients. Crit Care Med 2007;35:1530–5.
58. Garland A, Shaman Z, Baron J, et al. Physician-attributable differences in intensive care unit costs: a single-center study. Am J Respir Crit Care Med 2006;174:1206–10.
59. Scales DC, Laupacis A. Health technology assessment in critical care. Intensive Care Med 2007;33:2183–91.
60. Harvey S, Singer M. Managing critically ill patients with a pulmonary artery catheter. Br J Hosp Med (Lond) 2006;67:421–6.
61. Wiener RS, Welch HG. Trends in the use of the pulmonary artery catheter in the United States, 1993–2004. JAMA 2007;298:423–9.
62. Pronovost P, Needham D, Berenholtz S, et al. An intervention to decrease catheter-related bloodstream infections in the ICU. N Engl J Med 2006;355:2725–32.
63. Weiss CH, Moazed F, McEvoy CA, et al. Prompting physicians to address a daily checklist and process of care and clinical outcomes: a single-site study. Am J Respir Crit Care Med 2011.
64. Girard TD, Kress JP, Fuchs BD, et al. Efficacy and safety of a paired sedation and ventilator weaning protocol for mechanically ventilated patients in intensive care (Awakening and Breathing Controlled trial): a randomised controlled trial. Lancet 2008;371(9607):126–34.

65. Haynes AB, Weiser TG, Berry WR, et al. A surgical safety checklist to reduce morbidity and mortality in a global population. N Engl J Med 2009;360:491–9.

66. Dellinger RP, Carlet JM, Masur H, et al. Surviving Sepsis Campaign guidelines for management of severe sepsis and septic shock. Crit Care Med 2004;32:858–73.

67. Logan AC, Yank V, Stafford RS. Off-label use of recombinant factor VIIa in U.S. hospitals: analysis of hospital records. Ann Intern Med 2011;154:516–22.

68. Yank V, Tuohy CV, Logan AC, et al. Systematic review: benefits and harms of in-hospital use of recombinant factor VIIa for off-label indications. Ann Intern Med 2011;154:529–40.

69. Merlani P, Garnerin P, Diby M, et al. Quality improvement report: Linking guideline to regular feedback to increase appropriate requests for clinical tests: blood gas analysis in intensive care. BMJ 2001;323(7313):620–4.

70. Zimmerman JE, Alzola C, Von Rueden KT. The use of benchmarking to identify top performing critical care units: a preliminary assessment of their policies and practices. J Crit Care 2003;18:76–86.

71. McAlpine L, Cohen IL, Truckenbrod A. Reducing resource consumption through work redesign in a surgical intensive care unit: a multidisciplinary, protocol-based progressive care area. Heart Lung 2007;26:329–34.

72. Krieger BP, Ershowsky P, Spivack D. One year's experience with a noninvasively monitored intermediate care unit for pulmonary patients. JAMA 1990;264:1143–6.

73. Gracey DR, Hardy DC, Koenig GE. The chronic ventilator-dependent unit: a lower-cost alternative to intensive care. Mayo Clin Proc 2000;75:445–9.

74. Dasgupta A, Rice R, Mascha E, et al. Four-year experience with a unit for long-term ventilation (respiratory special care unit) at the Cleveland Clinic Foundation. Chest 1999;116:447–55.

75. Elpern E, Silver MR, Rosen RL, et al. The noninvasive respiratory care unit. Patterns of use and financial implications. Chest 1991;99:205–8.

76. Kahn JM, Benson NM, Appleby D, et al. Long-term acute care hospital utilization after critical illness. JAMA 2010;303:2253–9.

77. Kahn JM, Goss CH, Heagerty PJ, et al. Hospital volume and the outcomes of mechanical ventilation. N Engl J Med 2006;355:41–50.

78. Nathens AB, Jurkovich GJ, Maier RV, et al. Relationship between trauma center volume and outcomes. JAMA 2001;285:1164–71.

79. Phibbs CS, Bronstein JM, Buxton E, et al. The effects of patient volume and level of care at the hospital of birth on neonatal mortality. JAMA 1996;276:1054–9.

80. Hutchings A, Durand MA, Grieve R, et al. Evaluation of modernisation of adult critical care services in England: time series and cost effectiveness analysis. BMJ 2009;339:b4353.

81. Iwashyna TJ, Christie JD, Moody J, et al. The structure of critical care transfer networks. Med Care 2009;47:787–93.

82. Kahn JM, Asch RJ, Iwashyna TJ, et al. Physician attitudes toward regionalization of adult critical care: a national survey. Crit Care Med 2009;37:2149–54.

83. Kahn JM, Linde-Zwirble WT, Wunsch H, et al. Potential value of regionalized intensive care for mechanically ventilated medical patients. Am J Respir Crit Care Med 2008;177:285–91.

84. Cummings J, Krsek C, Vermoch K, et al. Intensive care unit telemedicine: review and consensus recommendations. Am J Med Qual 2007;22:239–50.

85. Thomas EJ, Lucke JF, Wueste L, et al. Association of telemedicine for remote monitoring of intensive care patients with mortality, complications, and length of stay. JAMA 2009;302:2671–8.

86. Morrison JL, Cai Q, Davis N, et al. Clinical and economic outcomes of the electronic intensive care unit: results from two community hospitals. Crit Care Med 2010;38: 2–8.
87. Lilly CM, Cody S, Zhao H, et al. Hospital mortality, length of stay, and preventable complications among critically ill patients before and after tele-ICU reengineering of critical care processes. JAMA 2011;305:2175–83.
88. Franzini L, Sail KR, Thomas EJ, et al. Costs and cost-effectiveness of a telemedicine intensive care unit program in 6 intensive care units in a large health care system. J Crit Care 2011;26:329.
89. Scales DC, Dainty K, Hales B, et al. A multifaceted intervention for quality improvement in a network of intensive care units: a cluster randomized trial. JAMA 2011; 305:363–372.

Economics of Mechanical Ventilation and Respiratory Failure

Colin R. Cooke, MD, MSc[a,b,*]

KEYWORDS

- Cost-effectiveness • Health expenditures • Health resources
- Health services research • Quality of life

EPIDEMIOLOGY, OUTCOMES, AND ECONOMIC BURDEN

Acute respiratory failure is a common and life-threatening consequence of a diverse group of diseases, including those that cause a failure of gas exchange, a failure of airway protection mechanisms, or the need for temporary respiratory support after general anesthesia.[1,2] For patients who have acute respiratory failure, mechanical ventilation (MV) provides the most common, definitive, and potentially life-saving therapy.

The use of MV is common in the United States and throughout the world and is increasing over time.[3,4] Mechanically ventilated patients now represent approximately 3% of all acute care hospitalizations and 30% of all intensive care unit (ICU) admissions.[1,2,5] In 2005, the estimated incidence in of invasive MV in the United States was 2.8 per 1000 population, representing over 700,000 patients who receive MV per year in the United States alone.[2] This incidence rate increases dramatically with age; patients over the age of 65 receive MV at rates that are 3 to 5 times the national average.[2]

Ventilated patients are at great risk of dying during the course of their illness and also have higher rates of long-term morbidity compared with non–mechanically ventilated ICU patients.[1,2] Approximately 30% to 40% of all patients who require MV die without ever being discharged.[1,2,6] Those who survive hospitalization more often confront frequent readmissions, are often left dependent upon others for their care owing to long-term disability or persistent need for respiratory support, and have significantly reduced life expectancies compared with nonventilated patients.[7–9]

Disclosure: Dr Cooke is supported by the Robert Wood Johnson Foundation Clinical Scholars program.

[a] Division of Pulmonary & Critical Care Medicine, University of Michigan, Ann Arbor, MI 48109, USA
[b] Center for Healthcare Outcomes & Policy, University of Michigan, Ann Arbor, MI 48109, USA
* Corresponding author. Center for Healthcare Outcomes & Policy, North Campus Research Complex, 2800 Plymouth Road, Building 520, Room 3141, Ann Arbor, MI 48109-2800.
E-mail address: cookecr@umich.edu

As a consequence of its high incidence, resource needs, and associated poor outcomes, MV is extraordinarily costly.[1,2,5,7] Although ventilated patients represent a small fraction of hospitalizations, they account for a disproportionate share of hospital days and costs. In 2005, the mean hospital length of stay for a ventilated patient was 14 days, representing 7% of all hospital days. In the same year, total hospital costs for care of an adult ventilated patient was $34,257.[2] When multiplied by the estimated 700,000 MV patients in the United States, this represents $27.0 billion or 12% of all hospital costs.[2] Patients older than 65 years account for more than half of MV expenditures.[2] As the elderly population increases rapidly and medical technology and management improve, the costs of MV to society will only increase.[3] Because of the expected growth in MV, it will likely be a major contributor to the unrelenting spending growth that now threatens Medicare's fiscal sustainability.[10,11] Reducing the costs of critical care in general, and MV in particular, is a major priority for providers, health system administrators, and payers and policymakers. It is, therefore, increasingly important to understand the costs and consequences of MV as a therapy aimed at reducing mortality and improving the health of critically ill patients.

This article reviews the body of literature examining the costs and cost effectiveness of invasive and noninvasive MV for the treatment of respiratory failure, highlights the clinical implications of this body of work, and suggests areas in this field in need of further research.

INCREMENTAL COSTS

The costs associated with MV play a central role in all economic analyses in critical care because patients receiving MV are not only common, but also costly. The majority of patients who require MV for respiratory failure require admission to an ICU, a location in the hospital that comes with significantly greater short-term fixed costs of care (**Fig. 1**).[2,5] Fixed costs are costs that are independent of patient throughput (ie, paid regardless of occupancy) such as staff salaries, utility payments, and other overhead.[12] Higher fixed costs in the ICU largely result from the greater nurse and other provider staffing and advanced support and monitoring equipment not available elsewhere. These costs account for 80% of total costs for a typical patient.[12,13] By definition, daily fixed ICU costs are the same for all ICU patients, but because ventilated patients occupy a large proportion of ICU beds and have longer ICU and hospital lengths of stay than nonventilated patients, they account for a disproportionate share of a hospital's total fixed costs. Mechanically ventilated patients also have greater variable costs. Variable costs are those that change owing to patient throughput and include pharmaceuticals, blood products, laboratory tests, and supplies required for patient care.[14] By nature of their greater severity of illness, ventilated patients consume more of these resources than nonventilated patients.[13,15,16] In addition to higher average total daily costs (fixed plus variable), MV patients are at greater risk of incurring greater downstream costs from longer lengths of stay owing to complications of care. For example, nosocomial pneumonia,[17] catheter-related blood stream infections,[17,18] and gastrointestinal hemorrhage[19] occur more commonly in ventilated patients. Finally, survivors of MV have greater functional disability after hospital discharge than average ICU patients, which brings significant additional long-term costs to society.[8]

A recent study by Dasta and colleagues[5] examined the incremental costs of MV by comparing the total costs of care between ventilated and nonventilated patients. The authors examined billing claims from more than 50,000 ICU admissions in 2002 from a geographically diverse sample of 253 hospitals in the United States. In the sample, ventilated patients spent longer in the ICU than nonventilated patients (mean, 6.9 vs

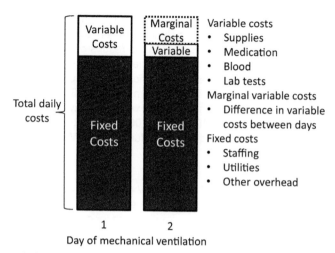

Fig. 1. Schematic illustrating the various components of total daily intensive care unit costs for a mechanically ventilated patient from the perspective of a hospital. Fixed daily costs represent 80% of total daily intensive care unit costs and include costs of equipment and overhead. Variable costs depend on the resources delivered to the patient and thus depend on patient throughput. Marginal variable costs represent the difference in variable cost between days, or ICU costs that might be saved by reducing duration of mechanical ventilation by 1 day. Examples of several important components of variable and fix cost are listed.

2.9 days) and had greater average ICU costs ($31,574 vs $12,931, 2003 $US). After adjusting for several patient and hospital differences, MV was the greatest predictor of daily ICU costs. The adjusted mean incremental daily cost of MV was $1522. When stratified by the day of ICU stay, mean incremental costs of MV were greatest on day 1 and declined the farther out a patient was from the day of admission.

Additional studies similarly demonstrate that MV patients have greater lengths of stay and costs than nonventilated patients, but together these studies have also led to the assumption that reducing the duration of MV for a patient could result in cost savings.[20,21] However, as suggest by several authors, this perception has several flaws worthy of note.[13,22,23] First, as exemplified by Dasta and associates,[5] most economic studies of MV compare total daily costs or total hospital costs between ventilated and nonventilated patients. Total costs are dominated by fixed costs that cannot be recovered by shortening hospital stay. Second, shortening the duration of MV may only exchange MV days for non-MV days; thus, any extra non-MV costs that result from early extubation must be factored into and against the cost savings attributed to any observed reduction in duration of MV. Third, because costs vary by day in the ICU, reducing a patient's duration of MV saves only the marginal costs of an additional day of MV (see **Fig. 1**), not the mean daily costs, which represents an average of high costs from early days in the ICU and lower costs from later days. Finally, extubating a ventilated patient does not mean that his or her costs will mirror those of a patient who never required ventilator support in the first place.[13,22]

Kahn and colleagues[13] addressed several of these flaws in an analysis of the costs of a day of MV. In their study, the authors examined fixed and variable costs of care for each day among 1778 mechanically ventilated patients at a single academic medical center. Instead of comparing separate ventilated with nonventilated groups, the authors compared costs within the same patients before and after extubation. The average ICU cost for each ventilated patient was $54,468, of which $10,516 were direct-variable costs (19.3%), defined as total costs less overhead, staff salary, and equipment costs (ie, variable costs). Similar to the results of Dasta and co-wrokers[5] and others,[24] the direct-variable costs were highest during the first 2 days in the ICU (day 1, $4000; day 2, $1000), decreased significantly after day 2 and were subsequently stable. Of the 902 patients surviving more than 3 days in the ICU, the direct-variable cost difference between the last ventilator day and first nonventilator day (marginal cost) was a trivial $106. This $106 represents the per-patient dollar amount a hospital could save by reducing the duration of MV for a patient by 1 day.

Implications of the Literature

Although reductions in ICU length of stay for MV patients have unpredictable effects on hospital economics,[13] studies that have assessed the impact of MV upon ICU length of stay may have several important implications for calculating costs in the ICU. First, approximately 80% of the total costs for mechanically ventilated ICU patients are composed of fixed costs, which cannot be reduced in the short term by reducing length of stay. Second, the ICU costs of care for mechanically ventilated patients are greatest in the first 2 days, followed by a rapid decline and a subsequent plateau. Thus, a reduction in the ICU length of stay for a MV patient occurs on the flat of the cost curve and may not uniformly reduce costs. Third, the costs of the last MV day are minimally higher than the first non-MV day, suggesting that reductions in the duration of MV will also result in nonuniform cost savings. Economic analyses of critical care therapies should, therefore, assess only the daily marginal, or variable, costs of a decrease in duration of MV or ICU stay, and not the average total daily costs. Otherwise, there is a risk of overestimating the costs that may be saved from reductions in duration of MV that result from the therapy itself under investigation.

COST EFFECTIVENESS
Critical Care

The field of critical care has been relatively slow to adopt high-quality economic evaluations of most therapies delivered in the ICU, and MV is no exception. Several authors reviewed the critical care economic literature published before 2002 and concluded that most published studies to date assessed costs of care without integrating outcome, or effectiveness, data.[15,25–29] Similarly, many studies that employed more sophisticated methods such as cost-effectiveness analysis to assess the economic impact of MV, failed to meet methodological standards for high-quality analysis.[28,29]

The authors of these reviews concluded that the paucity of high-quality economic analyses in critical care was attributable to the lack of critical care interventions proven effective and a lack of standards for the conduct of high-quality analyses. However, since these reviews were conducted there has been a surge in critical care therapies, including several strategies of MV, shown to improve patient outcomes.[30–32] In addition, in 2002 the American Thoracic Society published guidelines for the conduct of high-quality cost-effectiveness studies in critical care.[33] These 2 events may have helped to spur an increase in the number of published economic evaluations of critical care therapies.[34] The following sections highlight prior and more recent literature on the cost-effectiveness of several aspects of MV. Of note, throughout this review the term "cost effectiveness" is used to broadly refer to both traditional cost-effectiveness (cost per life saved) studies and cost-utility studies (cost per quality-adjusted life-year [QALY] gained).

Acute Respiratory Failure

Talmor and colleagues[29] recently published a systematic review that included several studies examining the cost effectiveness of MV in disease-specific populations. Their review identified 4 studies that examined MV for acute respiratory failure owing to pulmonary causes[35–38] and 1 study examining MV in the context of acute stroke.[39] The authors included these studies because they presented cost per QALY gained or cost per life-year gained incremental cost-effectiveness ratios. Since this systematic review was published, there has been 1 additional cost-effectiveness analysis of MV for acute respiratory failure published.[40]

The selected studies varied greatly in their target populations and their approach to determining the cost effectiveness of MV (**Table 1**). Three studies compared patients receiving MV with those who did not,[36,39,40] and 3 compared MV with withholding or withdrawing MV.[35,37,38] All of the studies were of low to moderate quality and analyzed costs from the perspective of the healthcare system.[29] Specifically, studies that received lower quality ratings were less likely to discount costs and QALYs,[35,36,40] were less likely to perform sensitivity analyses,[35,36,40] or did not include any costs after hospital discharge.[40]

The reported cost effectiveness of MV also varied considerably across studies. After inflation to 2011 $USD, the cost per life-year gained for MV in the 2 studies reporting this outcome varied from to $53,900[39] to $288,600.[35] Patients who received MV for _Pneumocystis carinii_ pneumonia in the setting of HIV infection before availability of antiretroviral medications had the highest cost per life-year gained ($288,600). The reported cost per QALY ranged from $26,000[36] to $175,000[35]; when inflated to 2011 costs, these ratios varied from $40,000 to $249,700. Reported cost-effectiveness ratios in these studies varied substantially by the underlying disease, severity of illness, and age in the target population.

Two studies explicitly examined the relationship between cost per QALY and age or severity of underlying disease.[37,38] Using a previously validated prognostic model for death,[41] Hamel and colleagues[37] stratified the calculation of cost-effectiveness ratios for 1005 patients receiving MV for pneumonia or acute respiratory distress syndrome by the likelihood of death within 2 months of acute respiratory failure diagnosis. The authors divided patients into high-risk, medium-risk, and low-risk (≤50%, 51%–70%, or >70% probability of surviving 2 months, respectively) and determined cost-effectiveness ratios for each group. The incremental cost-effectiveness ($US costs/QALY [2011]) were $40,000, $60,700, and $153,000 in the low-, medium-, and high-risk groups, respectively.

A second study by Hamel and colleagues[38] examined how the cost-effectiveness varied across 3 age groups (<65, 65–74, ≥75 years) in the same target population. Using the same prognostic model as in their prior study, the authors stratified results by the likelihood of death at 2 months (≤50% or >50%).[41] Within each age group costs per QALY among higher risk patients were greater (**Table 2**). However, the relationship between age and the cost-effectiveness ratios depended on the patient's predicted risk of death. Among low-risk patients, MV was less cost-effective among older patients, but among high-risk patients, MV was more cost-effective among older patients. The authors suggested that this somewhat paradoxical finding was attributable to the fact that 1-year survival among all high-risk patients was extremely low and therefore costs were driven primarily by the initial hospitalization costs. These costs were considerably higher among younger patients, perhaps because of earlier withdrawal of care among older patients.

Table 1
Summary of cost-effectiveness studies examining invasive MV for acute respiratory failure

References	Target Population	Intervention/ Comparator	Perspective/Time Horizon	Study Quality[a]	Cost Effectiveness, $/QALY (year)[b]
Wachter et al[35] (1995)	*Pneumocystis carinii* pneumonia (AIDS) and acute respiratory failure	MV/MV withheld (death)	Healthcare/NA	3	Cost/life-year $174,781 (1991) $416,800 (2011)
Anon et al[36] (1999)	Ventilated patients for COPD exacerbation on long-term oxygen	MV/No MV	Healthcare/lifetime	2	$26,283–$44,602 (1993) $53,700–$91,100 (2011)
Mayer et al[39] (2000)	Patients age >39 yrs ventilated for stroke	MV/No MV	Healthcare/lifetime	5	$174,200 (1996) $306,800 (2011)
Hamel et al[37] (2000)	Acute respiratory failure (ARDS or pneumonia) with APACHE II > 9	MV/MV withheld	Healthcare/lifetime	4	$29,000–$110,000 (1998) $48,000–$182,000 (2011)
Hamel et al[38] (2001)	Acute respiratory failure (ARDS or pneumonia) with APACHE II > 9	MV/MV withheld	Healthcare/lifetime	4	$32,000–$130,000 (1998) $53,000–$215,000 (2011)
Linko et al[40] (2010)	ICU patients requiring invasive or noninvasive ventilation	MV/no MV	Inpatient/lifetime	2	$1,936 (2008)[c] $2,142 (2011)

Abbreviations: APACHE, Acute Physiology Assessment and Chronic Health Evaluation; ARDS, acute respiratory distress syndrome; COPD, chronic obstructive pulmonary disease; NA, not available.

[a] Study quality (range, 1–7; higher is better) as reported by Talmor et al or Tufts Cost-Effectiveness Registry (https://research.tufts-nemc.org/cear4/default.aspx).

[b] Costs reported in original publication and inflated to 2011 $US using the medical portion of the Consumer Price Index.

[c] Costs in Euros converted to $US based on 12/2008 exchange rate of $1.3919 per Euro. Does not reflect the incremental cost-effectiveness ratio, rather only reports hospital costs/QALY among survivors.

Table 2						
Summary of the cost-effectiveness ratios for MV by risk of death and age reported by Hamel et al[38]						
	Low Risk (>50% Estimated Survival)			High Risk (<51% Estimated Survival)		
Year	Age <65	Age 56–74	Age ≥75	Age <65	Age 56–74	Age ≥75
1998	$32,000	$44,000	$46,000	$130,000	$100,000	$96,000
2011[a]	$53,000	$72,800	$76,100	$215,100	$165,500	$158,900

[a] Inflated to 2011 $US using the medical portion of the Consumer Price Index.

Implications of the Literature

There are several important conclusions that arise from these studies. First, based on current standards for cost effectiveness, MV is considered cost effective in the majority of patients.[42] Second, the cost effectiveness of MV in these studies varies quite noticeably owing to differences in the comparison group for MV, time horizon, and the calculation of costs. For example, several studies accrued QALYs over the lifetime without assessing associated lifetime costs, thereby biasing the results toward a higher level of cost effectiveness and lower ratios of cost per QALY).[36,40] In addition, several studies examined only empiric data from MV patients and hence, do not estimate the incremental costs were the patient not intubated, an approach that therefore fails to examine the cost effectiveness of the decision to ventilate a patient.[35,36,39,40] Finally, heterogeneity in cost-effectiveness estimates also depends largely on the underlying population, including the cause of respiratory failure, the risk of short-term death, and age. MV is highly cost effective in younger patients and those at lower risk of death, but less so for older sicker patients by most standards.[42]

PROLONGED MV

An important and growing subset of mechanically ventilated patients is the group who experience prolonged MV (PMV). PMV is variably defined in the literature ranging from 2 or more days to 21 or more days of MV,[43] although MV for at least 6 hours per day for 21 days or longer has gained the most traction among the critical care community.[44] Approximately 5% to 10% of all patients who require MV for acute respiratory failure require PMV.[43,45] Patients with PMV experience high 1-year mortality rates, functional and cognitive impairments, and report poor quality of life.[43,45]

Economic Burden

The costs of care for this patient population are enormous and have been quantified by several investigators. According to Medicare statistics in 2005, per-inpatient charges for PMV patients exceed those of patients with sepsis, myocardial infarction, or gastrointestinal bleeding.[46] Median per-inpatient costs are estimated to be $60,000 for patients with 4 or more days of MV[47,48] and can exceed a mean of $200,000 per patient with 21 or more days of MV.[49] When combined with the additional costs of hospital readmissions, outpatient costs, long-term care, skilled nursing stays, and home health services often required for this population, the cost of care per independently functioning survivor at 1 year can exceed $3.5 million.[49]

Cost Effectiveness

Although several studies have examined the costs or cost effectiveness of ongoing care for patients with a prolonged ICU stay,[50–53] many of whom require MV, only 2

Table 3
Summary of cost-effectiveness studies examining PMV

Reference	Target Population	Intervention	Comparator	Cost Effectiveness $/QALY[a]	Cost Effectiveness $/Life-Year
Cohen et al[54] (1993)	ICU patients (age ≥80) requiring ≥3 days of MV	MV	None	NA	$123,900 (1992) $271,800 (2011)
Cox et al[55] (2007)	ICU patients requiring ≥21 days of MV	MV ≥21 days	Withdrawal of ventilation (vented ≥7 but <21 days)	$82,400 (2005) $103,100 (2011)	$55,500 (2005) $69,500 (2011)

Abbreviation: NA, not available.
[a] Costs inflated to 2011 $US using the medical portion of the Consumer Price Index.

published studies specifically estimated the cost effectiveness of MV in isolation among patients requiring PMV.[54,55] The populations, intervention and comparisons, and the primary results for these 2 studies are reported in **Table 3**.

Cohen and associates[54] performed an empiric analysis of total hospitalization costs and years of life saved among 45 elderly patients (age ≥80) requiring MV for 3 or more days in a tertiary-care, university-affiliated hospital. Using the accrued hospital costs beyond 3 days for all patients and the life expectancy for survivors, the authors determined that the incremental cost of MV per life-year gained was $123,900 (1992 $US). In a post hoc analysis, they generated a prognostic index defined as age in years (*A*) + duration of MV in days (*D*). Nearly 40% of the total charges accrued by the entire study cohort occurred among the 22 patients when *A* + *D* exceeded 100. The costs of MV per life-year gained when *A* + *D* exceeded 100 was $300,800. Interestingly, the study only included incremental hospitalization costs suggesting that had total lifetime costs been included, costs per life-year gained would be far greater.

In a more comprehensive analysis, Cox and colleagues[55] used decision analysis and Markov modeling to determine the cost effectiveness of PMV. The authors first developed a decision tree that accounted for the decision to continue MV for 21 or more days (vs withdrawal of MV after 7 days but before 21 days), and the likelihood of surviving to hospital discharge. Patients who survived to hospital discharge were entered into a complex Markov process that modeled their likelihood of returning to full health, hospital readmission, transfer to skilled nursing or other long-term, acute-care, or rehabilitation facility, or death. Associated costs for each of these locations or health states and the associated healthcare costs for each were accrued in the modeling process and informed by a large prospective cohort of 813 ICU patients who received MV for 48 hours or longer.[47] Additional inputs for the model were taken from the medical literature.

PMV was cost effective under a variety of circumstances, but varied by age and risk of death. For the base-case patient (65-year-old of average race and gender), PMV had an incremental cost of $82,400 per QALY gained ($103,100 in 2011 $US); however, this ratio varied dramatically depending on the patient's age. Incremental costs per QALY gained for an 18-year-old was $14,289 (2005) compared with more than $206,000 (2005) for an 85-year-old. A 65-year-old with at least a 50% chance of death at 1 year had an incremental cost of $101,800 per QALY gained compared with $60,900 for the same patient with less than a 50% chance of death at 1 year. Although results were sensitive to estimates of acute hospitalization costs as well as the rates of readmission, the incremental cost per QALY for the base case remained above $100,000 over the range of probable model inputs.

Implications of the Literature

The results of these 2 PMV cost-effectiveness studies have several important implications. First, for the average patient who requires PMV, PMV is cost effective by modern standards.[42] However, as the age of the individual increases, this therapy becomes less cost effective by traditionally accepted norms.[42] For example, patients who are require PMV at 45 years of age have a incremental cost-effectiveness ratio of approximately $75,000 (2011) per QALY compared with more than $206,000 (2011 dollars) for an 85-year-old. Lower cost effectiveness among the elderly is concerning given current population projections. As the US population ages, there is potential for a massive influx of patients who require PMV. By 2020, the annual volume of PMV patients (>96 hours) is expected to exceed 600,000 patients.[56] To confront this impending burden of PMV, hospitals, payers, policymakers, and society must develop strategies to improve the cost effectiveness of PMV to help increase the likelihood that scarce resources are put to their most efficient use to achieve the highest level of expected benefit relative to costs that are expended.

One strategy is to target and improve the relatively poor quality of life for patients with PMV.[55] Because the cost effectiveness of PMV is highly dependent on the quality of life of PMV, small improvements in the quality of life may dramatically alter the cost effectiveness of this therapy.[55] Several options, such as dedicated post-ICU clinics, structured outpatient rehabilitation programs, and disease management programs, offer ways to potentially improve the quality of life of survivors of PMV and make this therapy more cost effective. Efficacy studies for some of these therapies exist,[57–59] and several additional studies are underway.[60–63]

Hospitals have already discovered that 1 potential way to decrease the costs of PMV in the acute care phase is to provide care for these patients in alternative settings outside of the ICU. For example, a large percentage of PMV patients are transferred to long-term acute-care facilities during their initial episode of MV.[64] By discharging resource-intensive patients early in their care, hospitals can cost shift the care of these patients to other facilities.[65,66] However, we know little about how such facilities impact the societal costs of their care. By virtue of their economies of scale and greater specialization of services, long-term acute-care facilities may reduce length of stay or hospital readmissions and improve the costs and outcomes of care for PMV patients. Reduced nurse and physician staffing at such facilities may also contribute to lower costs of care.[67] However, these potential benefits may also be associated with potential harm, because lower levels of nurse and physician staffing may lead to worse outcomes for this population,[68] and the absence of diagnostic and therapeutic resources usually present in acute care facilities may delay the definitive management of illness these patients. Long-term acute-care facilities are only one of several post-ICU locations where patients with PMV may receive care. Intermediate care units (ie, step-down units), skilled nursing facilities, rehabilitation facilities, and even home are all potential options, each potentially less costly than the ICU. These issues highlight the need for further research studying how alternative locations of care might improve the cost effectiveness of PMV.

VENTILATOR MANAGEMENT STRATEGIES
Is There a Need to Examine the Cost Effectiveness of Ventilator Management?

Very few authors have examined the economic aspects of different management strategies of MV owing to the absence of demonstrated effectiveness. Traditionally, investigators reserve cost-effectiveness analysis for therapies that either improve patient outcomes, or are less costly relative to standard therapy. Several recent meta-analyses examining the effectiveness of different approaches to MV have failed to show benefit and thus are unlikely candidates for such analysis.[69] These studies have largely been limited to patients with acute lung injury (ALI), because this patient population characteristically requires the most aggressive and nuanced ventilator management of any hospitalized patient. For example, beyond standard of care, several randomized, controlled studies failed to show improvement in mortality for recruitment maneuvers,[69] a recent meta-analyses failed to show improvement in mortality for inhaled nitric oxide,[70] and an additional meta-analysis failed to show improvement in mortality for most, but not all, patients treated with prone positioning for refractory hypoxemia.[71]

There are several MV management strategies that do seem to improve survival among select patients with ALI. These include ventilation with lower tidal volumes,[30,72] higher levels of positive end expiratory pressure,[31] and high-frequency oscillatory ventilation.[32] Although not traditionally thought of as a strategy of MV, one recent study also suggested that extracorporeal membrane oxygenation may be a cost-effective approach to improving mortality among patients with acute respiratory distress syndrome and refractory hypoxemia.[73]

Cost Effectiveness of Low Tidal Volume Ventilation

Of the effective ventilator management strategies described, only low-tidal volume ventilation has been subjected to a formal cost-effectiveness analysis. Cooke and colleagues[74] designed a simulation informed by empiric data to assess the cost effectiveness of delivering lung-protective ventilation to patients with ALI. The authors compared costs and consequences of delivering MV with a tidal volume of 6 cc/kg to a more traditional tidal volume of 12 cc/kg. Both short- and long-term healthcare costs informed by the literature were accrued over the lifetime of each patient.

The primary results demonstrated that the 6 cc/kg tidal volume strategy was highly cost effective. For the base case, the incremental cost of the 6 cc/kg strategy was $11,690 (2008) per QALY gained and $22,566 (2008) per life saved, compared with the 12 cc/kg strategy. The results of this analysis were not sensitive to the vast majority of variable inputs. A probabilistic sensitivity analysis indicated that 98.9% of all simulations, where model inputs were randomly drawn from their distribution, maintained an incremental cost per QALY of less than $50,000 (2008).

In a secondary analysis, the authors evaluated the cost effectiveness of hypothetical ICU-based intervention aimed to improve adherence to delivering 6 cc/kg to all patients with ALI. The analysis demonstrated that a sizeable investment in improving adherence to 6 cc/kg at the ICU level would remain cost effective. For example, ICUs could invest up to $3556 (2008) per patient with ALI into an ICU-wide intervention to improving their adherence to low tidal volumes by 15% (from 70% to 85% of patients). The authors concluded that 6 cc/kg was a cost-effective MV strategy and is worth considerable investment by ICUs and hospitals to ensure that patients receive this therapy.

Implications of the Literature

There are several important implications that result from these studies discussed. First, delivering low tidal volume ventilation is cost effective. Hospitals should be willing to invest a considerable amount in the development of a program that ensures all patients with ALI receive low tidal volume ventilation. Second, there several effective ventilator management strategies that are in need of formal cost-effectiveness analysis, including high-frequency oscillatory ventilation, and ventilation with high levels of positive end-expiratory pressure. The incremental costs of delivering alternative modes of ventilation to a patient who is already receiving traditional MV are likely small suggesting that these therapies may potentially be cost effective when used in the appropriate population deemed most likely to benefit. This is exemplified by the cost-effectiveness analysis of low tidal volume discussed.[74]

NONINVASIVE MV

Noninvasive ventilation (NIV) represents an appealing alternative to invasive MV in certain populations from the perspective of considering ways to minimize ways to minimize the costs of care for patients with acute respiratory failure without compromising clinical effectiveness. Specifically, NIV provides ventilator support using a nasal or facemask interface between the ventilator and patient. By averting an artificial airway, patients who use NIV can often avoid intravenous sedation and costly complications, such as ventilator-associated pneumonia, sinusitis, and line sepsis.[75,76] Avoiding these consequences of intubation reduces length of ICU and hospital stay that, as discussed, are tightly linked to costs of care. Although most traditional ventilators can provide noninvasive support, NIV can be provided by a much less costly portable machine, and can often be safely delivered in less resource-intensive settings, such as outside of the ICU on the general wards.[76]

In addition to its potential for cost savings, NIV is highly effective in many clinical settings. Although indicated for several causes of acute respiratory failures, NIV has been most consistently shown to improve outcomes among patients acute respiratory acidosis caused by an exacerbation of chronic obstructive pulmonary disease (COPD). In this population, at least 4 meta-analyses demonstrate better outcomes for NIV compared with standard therapy.[77–80] For example, 1 recent meta-analysis concluded that NIV reduces hospital length of stay in this population by approximately 5 days, reduced the absolute rates of endotracheal intubation by 28%, and decreased in-hospital mortality by 10%.[78]

Cost Effectiveness

In contrast with the large number of studies demonstrating better outcomes for NIV in acute respiratory failure owing to COPD, relatively few studies have performed formal economic analyses of this therapy. Keenan and colleagues[81] conducted an economic evaluation to estimate the potential cost savings of managing patients with severe COPD exacerbation (symptoms, elevated PCO_2, pH <7.35) with NIV compared with standard care (antibiotics, bronchodilators, steroids, and oxygen). The authors developed a theoretical decision model informed by a meta-analysis and comprehensive literature search to populate the parameters of their model. The analysis assumed that patients were admitted to an intermediate care unit for observation, or NIV and required 2 to 4 hours per day of respiratory therapy support. All hospital costs were accounted for and included direct costs such as supplies, equipment, power, capital (ventilators), and overhead costs. Because the perspective of the analysis was the hospital, the authors did not include any postdischarge costs and did not assess long-term quality of life and, therefore, were unable to calculate cost per QALY gained. Instead, the primary outcome of the analysis was cost per COPD patient saved.

The primary results of the study by Keenan and associates demonstrated that management of COPD patients with hypercapneic respiratory failure using NIV was cost saving. Hospital costs of care for the NIV group was $7211 (1996 $Can) compared with $10,455 (1996 $Can) for the standard group, a cost savings of $3244 (1996 $Can) or $4170 (2011 $US) per admission. Importantly, this cost savings was maintained when all patients were assumed to be admitted to the ICU instead of an intermediate care unit (cost savings of $3044 $Can), and if 24-hour respiratory therapy support was required (cost savings of $1290 $Can). Given the well-demonstrated, superior outcomes associated with NIV, the authors concluded that NIV was a "dominant" strategy, because it was deemed to be more effective and less costly relative to the alternative.

More recently, Plant and colleagues[82] conducted a cost-effectiveness analysis of ward-based NIV for acute exacerbations of COPD. In their analysis, the authors collected detailed cost data during the conduct of a randomized controlled trial in 14 centers in the United Kingdom. During the parent study, 236 patients with acute respiratory failure secondary to COPD (pH <7.35, respiratory rate >23) were randomized to standard therapy (oxygen, bronchodilators, steroids, antibiotics) or standard therapy plus NIV. NIV was primarily delivered on the wards, not in the ICU. The authors collected highly detailed hospital-based costs. Patients in the NIV strategy had lower hospital mortality and reduced costs. The incremental cost of NIV was approximately −$1064 per death avoided, indicating a dominant strategy. The vast majority of these cost savings were attributable to avoidance of care in the ICU.

Recognizing that NIV allows patient with COPD exacerbations to avoid care in more resource-intensive settings such as the ICU, Tuggey and colleagues[83] sought to determine whether NIV could prevent the need for hospitalization. The authors identified 13 patients from a single center in the United Kingdom who were admitted frequently for COPD exacerbations, tolerated NIV in the past, and were given home noninvasive ventilators. Hospital, outpatient, and equipment costs and consequences of care for the patients incurred the year after home NIV use were compared with those incurred in the year after NIV use. In the period before home NIV, patients had fewer hospital admissions, days in the hospital, ICU admissions, and outpatient appointments. This resulted in a cost-savings of approximately $12,320 (2000) per patient.

Implications of the Literature

These 3 studies suggest that NIV is a potentially cost-saving therapy when used for severe COPD exacerbations. However, these findings may not generalize to countries other than Canada or the United Kingdom. As highlighted by the 3 studies, patients requiring NIV in the United Kingdom are usually treated outside of the ICU and those in Canada are often managed in intermediate care units. The economic benefits of NIV may be less in hospitals where it is delivered in the ICU, as is the case in the United States and many European countries. As providers become more comfortable with managing NIV and the patients who require it, they may slowly shift the care for these patients to the ward, a phenomena that is already occurring.[84] Differences in staffing for NIV between countries may also challenge the generalizability of these studies. Nurses who managed NIV patients in the UK study required minimal additional time to care for NIV patients (<30 minutes). In the United States and Canada, respiratory therapists assume this responsibility and, as shown by Keenan et and co-workers,[81] the cost savings can decrease considerably as staffing requirements increase. Despite these limitations, NIV holds great economic promise as it is one of the very few effective critical care therapies that are cost saving.

SUMMARY

MV is the best life-sustaining treatment option for most patients with respiratory failure, but comes with considerable additional costs. Quantitating these excess costs is challenging and requires considering how MV fits into broader costs of ICU care. Although the costs of MV are high, the majority of patients who receive MV survive their illness and gain significant quality years of life that would have been lost without its use placing MV among the few cost-effective therapies in critical care. However, the cost effectiveness of MV is highly dependent on a patient's cause of respiratory failure, risk of death, and age. NIV of patients with COPD is cost saving whereas, NIV of older patients, and those at greater risk of death during their ICU stay, is much less cost effective. Because MV often prevents immediate death, providers will continue to offer it even to those with the lowest chance of benefit.[85,86] As we aim to improve the cost-effectiveness of MV, we should not solely focus on whom to ventilate, but rather on how we can better ventilate, and how we can improve the outcomes of MV and quality of life among those who survive MV.

ACKNOWLEDGMENTS
The author thanks Theodore J. Iwashyna for his helpful comments on an earlier draft of this manuscript.

REFERENCES

1. Esteban A, Anzueto A, Frutos F, et al. Characteristics and outcomes in adult patients receiving mechanical ventilation: a 28-day international study. JAMA 2002;287:345–55.
2. Wunsch H, Linde-Zwirble WT, Angus DC, et al. The epidemiology of mechanical ventilation use in the United States. Crit Care Med 2010;38:1947–53.
3. Needham DM, Bronskill SE, Calinawan JR, et al. Projected incidence of mechanical ventilation in Ontario to 2026: preparing for the aging baby boomers. Crit Care Med 2005;33:574–9.
4. Carson SS, Cox CE, Holmes GM, et al. The changing epidemiology of mechanical ventilation: a population-based study. J Intensive Care Med 2006;21:173–82.
5. Dasta JF, McLaughlin TP, Mody SH, et al. Daily cost of an intensive care unit day: the contribution of mechanical ventilation. Crit Care Med 2005;33:1266–71.
6. Luhr OR, Karlsson M, Thorsteinsson A, et al. The impact of respiratory variables on mortality in non-ARDS and ARDS patients requiring mechanical ventilation. Intensive Care Med 2000;26:508–17.
7. Wunsch H, Guerra C, Barnato AE, et al. Three-year outcomes for Medicare beneficiaries who survive intensive care. JAMA 2010;303:849–56.
8. Barnato AE, Albert SM, Angus DC, et al. Disability among elderly survivors of mechanical ventilation. Am J Respir Crit Care Med 2011;183:1037–42.
9. Desai SV, Law TJ, Needham DM. Long-term complications of critical care. Crit Care Med 2011;39:371–9.
10. Cooper LM, Linde-Zwirble WT. Medicare intensive care unit use: analysis of incidence, cost, and payment. Crit Care Med 2004;32:2247–53.
11. Orszag PR, Ellis P. The challenge of rising health care costs: a view from the congressional budget office. N Engl J Med 2007;357:1793–5.

12. Roberts RR, Frutos PW, Ciavarella GG, et al. Distribution of variable vs fixed costs of hospital care. JAMA 1999;281:644–9.
13. Kahn JM, Rubenfeld GD, Rohrbach J, et al. Cost savings attributable to reductions in intensive care unit length of stay for mechanically ventilated patients. Med Care 2008;46:1226–33.
14. Rossi C, Simini B, Brazzi L, et al. Variable costs of ICU patients: a multicenter prospective study. Intensive Care Med 2006;32:545–52.
15. Noseworthy TW, Konopad E, Shustack A, et al. Cost accounting of adult intensive care: methods and human and capital inputs. Crit Care Med 1996;24:1168–72.
16. Ezzie ME, Aberegg SK, O'Brien JM Jr. Laboratory testing in the intensive care unit. Crit Care Clin 2007;23:435–65.
17. Vincent JL, Rello J, Marshall J, et al. International study of the prevalence and outcomes of infection in intensive care units. JAMA 2009;302:2323–9.
18. Warren DK, Zack JE, Elward AM, et al. Nosocomial primary bloodstream infections in intensive care unit patients in a nonteaching community medical center: a 21-month prospective study. Clin Infect Dis 2001;33:1329–35.
19. Cook DJ, Fuller HD, Guyatt GH, et al. Risk factors for gastrointestinal bleeding in critically ill patients. Canadian Critical Care Trials Group. N Engl J Med 1994;330:377–81.
20. Ely EW, Baker AM, Dunagan DP, et al. Effect on the duration of mechanical ventilation of identifying patients capable of breathing spontaneously. N Engl J Med 1996;335:1864–9.
21. Schweickert WD, Gehlbach BK, Pohlman AS, et al. Daily interruption of sedative infusions and complications of critical illness in mechanically ventilated patients. Crit Care Med 2004;32:1272–6.
22. Kahn JM. Understanding economic outcomes in critical care. Curr Opin Crit Care 2006;12:399–404.
23. Luce JM, Rubenfeld GD. Can health care costs be reduced by limiting intensive care at the end of life? Am J Respir Crit Care Med 2002;165:750–4.
24. Rapoport J, Teres D, Zhao Y, et al. Length of stay data as a guide to hospital economic performance for ICU patients. Med Care 2003;41:386–97.
25. Chalfin DB, Cohen IL, Lambrinos J. The economics and cost-effectiveness of critical care medicine. Intensive Care Med 1995;21:952–61.
26. Gyldmark M. A review of cost studies of intensive care units: problems with the cost concept. Crit Care Med 1995;23:964–72.
27. Heyland DK, Guyatt G, Cook DJ, et al. Frequency and methodologic rigor of quality-of-life assessments in the critical care literature. Crit Care Med 1998;26:591–8.
28. Pines JM, Fager SS, Milzman DP. A review of costing methodologies in critical care studies. J Crit Care 2002;17:181–6.
29. Talmor D, Shapiro N, Greenberg D, et al. When is critical care medicine cost-effective? A systematic review of the cost-effectiveness literature. Crit Care Med 2006;34:2738–47.
30. Ventilation with lower tidal volumes as compared with traditional tidal volumes for acute lung injury and the acute respiratory distress syndrome. The Acute Respiratory Distress Syndrome Network. N Engl J Med 2000;342:1301–8.
31. Briel M, Meade M, Mercat A, et al. Higher vs lower positive end-expiratory pressure in patients with acute lung injury and acute respiratory distress syndrome: systematic review and meta-analysis. JAMA 2010;303:865–73.

32. Sud S, Sud M, Friedrich JO, et al. High frequency oscillation in patients with acute lung injury and acute respiratory distress syndrome (ARDS): systematic review and meta-analysis. BMJ 2010;340:c2327.

33. Understanding costs and cost-effectiveness in critical care. report from the second American Thoracic Society workshop on outcomes research. Am J Respir Crit Care Med 2002;165:540–50.

34. Tufts Cost-Effectiveness Analysis Registry. Available at: https://research.tufts-nemc.org/cear4/default.aspx. Accessed June, 2011.

35. Wachter RM, Luce JM, Safrin S, et al. Cost and outcome of intensive care for patients with AIDS, Pneumocystis carinii pneumonia, and severe respiratory failure. JAMA 1995;273:230–5.

36. Anon JM, Garcia de Lorenzo A, Zarazaga A, et al. Mechanical ventilation of patients on long-term oxygen therapy with acute exacerbations of chronic obstructive pulmonary disease: prognosis and cost-utility analysis. Intensive Care Med 1999;25:452–7.

37. Hamel MB, Phillips RS, Davis RB, et al. Outcomes and cost-effectiveness of ventilator support and aggressive care for patients with acute respiratory failure due to pneumonia or acute respiratory distress syndrome. Am J Med 2000;109:614–20.

38. Hamel MB, Phillips RS, Davis RB, et al. Are aggressive treatment strategies less cost-effective for older patients? The case of ventilator support and aggressive care for patients with acute respiratory failure. J Am Geriatr Soc 2001;49:382–90.

39. Mayer SA, Copeland D, Bernardini GL, et al. Cost and outcome of mechanical ventilation for life-threatening stroke. Stroke 2000;31:2346–53.

40. Linko R, Suojaranta-Ylinen R, Karlsson S, et al. One-year mortality, quality of life and predicted life-time cost-utility in critically ill patients with acute respiratory failure. Crit Care 2010;14:R60.

41. Knaus WA, Harrell FE Jr, Lynn J, et al. The SUPPORT prognostic model. Objective estimates of survival for seriously ill hospitalized adults. Study to understand prognoses and preferences for outcomes and risks of treatments. Ann Intern Med 1995;122:191–203.

42. Braithwaite RS, Meltzer DO, King JT Jr, et al. What does the value of modern medicine say about the $50,000 per quality-adjusted life-year decision rule? Med Care 2008;46:349–56.

43. Nelson JE, Cox CE, Hope AA, et al. Chronic critical illness. Am J Respir Crit Care Med 2010;182:446–54.

44. MacIntyre NR, Epstein SK, Carson S, et al. Management of patients requiring prolonged mechanical ventilation: report of a NAMDRC consensus conference. Chest 2005;128:3937–54.

45. Carson SS, Bach PB. The epidemiology and costs of chronic critical illness. Crit Care Clin 2002;18:461–76.

46. Centers for Medicare and Medicaid Services. Medicare provider analysis and review: long-term care hospitals. Available at: http://www.cms.hhs.gov. Accessed June 12, 2011.

47. Chelluri L, Mendelsohn AB, Belle SH, et al. Hospital costs in patients receiving prolonged mechanical ventilation: does age have an impact? Crit Care Med 2003;31:1746–51.

48. Zilberberg MD, Luippold RS, Sulsky S, et al. Prolonged acute mechanical ventilation, hospital resource utilization, and mortality in the United States. Crit Care Med 2008;36:724–30.

49. Unroe M, Kahn JM, Carson SS, et al. One-year trajectories of care and resource utilization for recipients of prolonged mechanical ventilation: a cohort study. Ann Intern Med 2010;153:167–75.

50. Becker GJ, Strauch GO, Saranchak HJ. Outcome and cost of prolonged stay in the surgical intensive care unit. Arch Surg 1984;119:1338–42.
51. Fakhry SM, Kercher KW, Rutledge R. Survival, quality of life, and charges in critically Ill surgical patients requiring prolonged ICU stays. J Trauma 1996;41:999–1007.
52. Heyland DK, Konopad E, Noseworthy TW, et al. Is it 'worthwhile' to continue treating patients with a prolonged stay (>14 days) in the ICU? An economic evaluation. Chest 1998;114:192–8.
53. Teno JM, Fisher E, Hamel MB, et al. Decision-making and outcomes of prolonged ICU stays in seriously ill patients. J Am Geriatr Soc 2000;48(5 Suppl):S70–4.
54. Cohen IL, Lambrinos J, Fein IA. Mechanical ventilation for the elderly patient in intensive care. Incremental changes and benefits. JAMA 1993;269:1025–9.
55. Cox CE, Carson SS, Govert JA, et al. An economic evaluation of prolonged mechanical ventilation. Crit Care Med 2007;35:1918–27.
56. Zilberberg MD, Shorr AF. Prolonged acute mechanical ventilation and hospital bed utilization in 2020 in the United States: implications for budgets, plant and personnel planning. BMC Health Serv Res 2008;8:242.
57. Martin UJ, Hincapie L, Nimchuk M, et al. Impact of whole-body rehabilitation in patients receiving chronic mechanical ventilation. Crit Care Med 2005;33:2259–65.
58. Kress JP. Clinical trials of early mobilization of critically ill patients. Crit Care Med 2009;37(10 Suppl):S442–7.
59. Schweickert WD, Pohlman MC, Pohlman AS, et al. Early physical and occupational therapy in mechanically ventilated, critically ill patients: a randomised controlled trial. Lancet 2009;373:1874–82.
60. National Institute of Mental Health. Preventing depression in people receiving mechanical ventilation in an intensive care unit. ClinicalTrials.gov. [Internet]. Bethesda (MD): National Library of Medicine (US). 2000. Available from: http://clinicaltrials.gov/ct2/show/NCT00872027. NLM Identifier: NCT00872027. Accessed June 8, 2011.
61. National Heart, Lung, and Blood Institute (NHLBI). Post-hospital case management to improve clinical outcomes in individuals requiring mechanical ventilation. ClinicalTrials.gov [Internet]. Bethesda (MD): National Library of Medicine (US). Available from:http://clinicaltrials.gov/ct2/show/NCT00149513. NLM Identifier: NCT00149513. Accessed cited June 8, 2011.
62. University Health Network, Toronto. Towards RECOVER: outcomes and needs assessment in intensive care unit (ICU) survivors of prolonged mechanical ventilation and their caregivers. ClinicalTrials.gov [Internet]. Bethesda (MD): National Library of Medicine (US). Available from:http://clinicaltrials.gov/ct2/show/NCT00896220. Accessed June 9, 2011.
63. Wake Forest University. Standardized rehabilitation for intensive care unit (ICU) patients with acute respiratory failure. In: ClinicalTrials.gov [Internet]. Bethesda (MD): National Library of Medicine (US). Available from: http://clinicaltrials.gov/ct2/show/NCT00976833. NLM Identifier:NCT00976833. Accessed June 8, 2011.
64. Kahn JM, Benson NM, Appleby D, et al. Long-term acute care hospital utilization after critical illness. JAMA 2010;303:2253–9.
65. Scheinhorn DJ, Artinian BM, Catlin JL. Weaning from prolonged mechanical ventilation. The experience at a regional weaning center. Chest 1994;105:534–9.
66. Seneff MG, Wagner D, Thompson D, et al. The impact of long-term acute-care facilities on the outcome and cost of care for patients undergoing prolonged mechanical ventilation. Crit Care Med 2000;28:342–50.
67. Liu K, Baseggio C, Wissoker D, et al. Long-term care hospitals under Medicare: facility-level characteristics. Health Care Financ Rev 2001;23:1–18.

68. Pronovost PJ, Angus DC, Dorman T, et al. Physician staffing patterns and clinical outcomes in critically ill patients: a systematic review. JAMA 2002;288:2151–62.
69. Pipeling MR, Fan E. Therapies for refractory hypoxemia in acute respiratory distress syndrome. JAMA 2010;304:2521–7.
70. Adhikari NK, Burns KE, Friedrich JO, et al. Effect of nitric oxide on oxygenation and mortality in acute lung injury: systematic review and meta-analysis. BMJ 2007;334: 779.
71. Sud S, Friedrich JO, Taccone P, et al. Prone ventilation reduces mortality in patients with acute respiratory failure and severe hypoxemia: systematic review and meta-analysis. Intensive Care Med 2010;36:585–99.
72. Petrucci N, Iacovelli W. Lung protective ventilation strategy for the acute respiratory distress syndrome. Cochrane Database Syst Rev 2007;3:CD003844.
73. Peek GJ, Mugford M, Tiruvoipati R, et al. Efficacy and economic assessment of conventional ventilatory support versus extracorporeal membrane oxygenation for severe adult respiratory failure (CESAR): a multicentre randomised controlled trial. Lancet 2009;374:1351–63.
74. Cooke CR, Kahn JM, Watkins TR, et al. Cost-effectiveness of implementing low-tidal volume ventilation in patients with acute lung injury. Chest 2009;136:79–88.
75. Davies JD, Gentile MA. What does it take to have a successful noninvasive ventilation program? Respir Care 2009;54:53–61.
76. Nava S, Hill N. Non-invasive ventilation in acute respiratory failure. Lancet 2009;374: 250–9.
77. Peter JV, Moran JL, Phillips-Hughes J, et al. Noninvasive ventilation in acute respiratory failure–a meta-analysis update. Crit Care Med 2002;30:555–62.
78. Keenan SP, Sinuff T, Cook DJ, et al. Which patients with acute exacerbation of chronic obstructive pulmonary disease benefit from noninvasive positive-pressure ventilation? A systematic review of the literature. Ann Intern Med 2003;138:861–70.
79. Lightowler JV, Wedzicha JA, Elliott MW, et al. Non-invasive positive pressure ventilation to treat respiratory failure resulting from exacerbations of chronic obstructive pulmonary disease: cochrane systematic review and meta-analysis. BMJ 2003;326: 185.
80. Quon BS, Gan WQ, Sin DD. Contemporary management of acute exacerbations of COPD: a systematic review and metaanalysis. Chest 2008;133:756–66.
81. Keenan SP, Gregor J, Sibbald WJ, et al. Noninvasive positive pressure ventilation in the setting of severe, acute exacerbations of chronic obstructive pulmonary disease: more effective and less expensive. Crit Care Med 2000;28:2094–102.
82. Plant PK, Owen JL, Parrott S, et al. Cost effectiveness of ward based non-invasive ventilation for acute exacerbations of chronic obstructive pulmonary disease: economic analysis of randomised controlled trial. BMJ 2003;326:956.
83. Tuggey JM, Plant PK, Elliott MW. Domiciliary non-invasive ventilation for recurrent acidotic exacerbations of COPD: an economic analysis. Thorax 2003;58:867–71.
84. Carlucci A, Delmastro M, Rubini F, et al. Changes in the practice of non-invasive ventilation in treating COPD patients over 8 years. Intensive Care Med 2003;29: 419–25.
85. Truog RD, Brock DW, Cook DJ, et al. Rationing in the intensive care unit. Crit Care Med 2006;34:958–63.
86. Kohn R, Rubenfeld GD, Levy MM, et al. Rule of rescue or the good of the many? An analysis of physicians' and nurses' preferences for allocating ICU beds. Intensive Care Med 2011;37:1210–7.

The Economics of Sepsis

Andrew N. Chalupka, BA[a], Daniel Talmor, MD, MPH[b,c,]*

KEYWORDS

- Sepsis • Bloodstream infection • Economics • Costs
- Cost-effectiveness

Sepsis, severe sepsis, and the systemic inflammatory response syndrome (SIRS) are among the most common reasons for admission to the intensive care unit (ICU). The global epidemiologic burden of sepsis is increasing for a variety of reasons, chief among them the aging population of developed countries. The financial burden of sepsis is also growing, due both to increasing fixed costs and to the development of expensive new drugs and technologies. Together these two phenomena lead to a significant economic impact that contributes to increasing strain on national and international health care resources.

To control costs, one must first understand their sources. This article describes the epidemiologic burden of sepsis, discusses the current literature on the economics of and costs associated with sepsis and its management, and examines the cost-effectiveness of sepsis interventions.

DEFINITIONS

Sepsis, a spectrum of systemic illness in response to severe infection, is an important cause of morbidity and mortality in critically ill patients. In 1991, the Society of Critical Care Medicine and the American College of Chest Physicians proposed standardized terminology providing a framework for the spectrum of illness surrounding sepsis. SIRS describes a dysregulated inflammatory response, regardless of origin, in which two or more of the following are present: body temperature greater than 38°C or less than 35°C, heart rate greater than 90 beats per minute, respiratory rate higher than 20 breaths per minute or one resulting in a $Paco_2$ below 32 mm Hg, and a white blood cell count of greater than $12,000/mm^3$ or less than $4000/mm^3$. When SIRS occurs in response to an infectious process, it is known as sepsis. Sepsis further complicated by organ failure, hypoperfusion, or hypotension is defined as severe sepsis. At the most

The authors have nothing to disclose.

[a] Harvard Medical School, 25 Shattuck Street, Boston, MA 02115, USA

[b] Department of Anesthesia, Critical Care, and Pain Medicine, Beth Israel Deaconess Medical Center, 1 Deaconess Road, CC-470, Boston, MA 02215, USA

[c] Department of Anesthesia, Harvard Medical School, 25 Shattuck Street, Boston, MA 02115, USA

* Corresponding author. Department of Anesthesia, Critical Care, and Pain Medicine, Beth Israel Deaconess Medical Center, 1 Deaconess Road, CC-470, Boston, MA 02215.

E-mail address: dtalmor@bidmc.harvard.edu

Crit Care Clin 28 (2012) 57–76

doi:10.1016/j.ccc.2011.09.003

0749-0704/12/$ – see front matter © 2012 Elsevier Inc. All rights reserved.

criticalcare.theclinics.com

serious end of the spectrum, septic shock describes severe sepsis accompanied by hypotension that persists despite adequate fluid resuscitation.[1] The use of older or alternative terminology, such as septicemia and bacteremia, still occurs in the literature on occasion. In instances where such literature is cited herein, the original terminology is preserved to avoid conflating separate clinical entities.

EPIDEMIOLOGY

The epidemiologic burden of sepsis in the United States is large and becoming larger. Analyzing hospital discharge data for 750 million hospitalizations nationwide, Martin and colleagues estimated that the population-adjusted incidence of sepsis increased by 8.7% per year between 1979 and 2000, from 82.7 cases per 100,000 population to 240.2 cases per 100,000 population.[2] Over this two-decade period, infections with gram-positive organisms leading to sepsis had the greatest increase (26.3% per year), accounting for 52.1% of sepsis cases by 2000. The proportion of patients developing organ failure doubled, from 16.8% in the period between 1979 and 1984 to 33.6% in the period between 1995 and 2000.

Significant demographic variation exists in the risk of developing sepsis.[2] For example, in the United States both blacks and other nonwhites experience higher rates of sepsis when compared to whites (relative risk [RR] = 1.89 for blacks and 1.90 for other nonwhites). From the standpoint of gender, the incidence of sepsis is higher in men (RR = 1.28), and the mean age at which men develop sepsis is younger (56.9 years old for men vs 62.1 years old for women). Elderly patients (65 years of age and older) accounted for 64.9% of sepsis cases between 1979 and 2002, and have a relative risk of developing sepsis of 13.1 compared with those under 65.[3] Case fatality rates also increase with age, as evidenced by a relative risk of death from sepsis that is 1.56 times greater among those older than the age of 65 compared with those younger than age 65.[3]

In the United States, sepsis accounts for a large mortality burden and is among the 10 leading causes of death.[4] Between 1999 and 2005, 6.0% of all deaths in the United States were associated with sepsis.[5] The number of deaths from sepsis nearly tripled between 1979 and 2000, from 43,579 to 120,491, reflecting the increase in incidence of sepsis. Survival improved, however, as reflected in a mortality rate among septic patients that declined from 27.8% in the period between 1979 and 1984 to 17.9% in the period between 1995 and 2000.[2]

The overall burden of severe sepsis is also increasing, in terms of both the number of patients who develop the syndrome and the extent and intensity of care that they require. In 1995, approximately 750,000 cases of severe sepsis occurred per year.[6] Among cases of severe sepsis, 51.1% receive ICU care, 11.1% receive care in a coronary care unit, and 6.2% were ventilated without receiving ICU care.[6] The proportion of severe sepsis patients among all sepsis patients increased by 1.7-fold between 1993 and 2003.[7] Over that time period, the incidence of hospitalization for severe sepsis increased from 64.7 to 134.6 per 100,000 population. The most frequently affected organ systems were the respiratory (28.4% of patients with severe sepsis), cardiovascular (25.3%), and renal (23.1%) systems. The proportion of patients with only one organ dysfunction decreased from 72.4% in 1993 to 58.2% in 2003, while the proportion of patients who had two, three, or four organ dysfunctions increased 1.3-, 1.9-, and 2.7-fold, respectively. Age-adjusted mortality rates due to severe sepsis increased at an annual rate of 5.6% from 30.3 deaths per 100,000 population in 1993 to 49.7 deaths per 100,000 population in 2003. However, case fatality dropped from 45.0% in 1993 to 37.7% in 2003, reflecting increased survival despite the increase in incidence.[7]

Sepsis also poses a significant burden of disease in pediatric patients. The incidence of severe sepsis in children is estimated to be 0.56 cases per 1000 children. The mean age of pediatric sepsis patients is 4.7 years. The incidence is highest in infants (5.16 cases per 1000 children), with 48% of cases in children younger than 1 year of age.[8]

Outside of the United States, sepsis imposes a formidable epidemiologic burden. In England, Wales, and Northern Ireland, the incidence of severe sepsis is 51 cases per 100,000 population.[9] In Spain, sepsis occurs in 114 of every 100,000 men.[10] In China, sepsis occurs in nearly 9% of all ICU admissions.[11] The incidence of severe sepsis in Taiwan is as high as 135 cases per 100,000 population.[12]

The incidence of and mortality associated with sepsis make it a global public health priority, yet national-level epidemiologic studies of sepsis exist almost exclusively for developed countries. A better understanding of the true global burden of sepsis would guide the design of health policy and the allocation of health care resources.[13] Adhikari and colleagues estimate that the global burden of sepsis is between 15 and 19 million cases per year, including approximately 5 million in East Asia, 4 million in South Asia, and 2 million in sub-Saharan Africa.[14]

Maternal sepsis and neonatal sepsis are of particular concern. The 2004 update to the World Health Organization's Global Burden of Disease (GBD) Report estimated that the worldwide incidence of maternal sepsis is 5.2 million cases per year.[15] Maternal sepsis is responsible for at least 75,000 deaths annually, disproportionately affecting low-income countries.[16] The same GBD report estimated that neonatal infections, including sepsis, account for 26% of deaths among neonates worldwide and 9% of deaths among children younger than the age of 5 years worldwide. National-level studies of neonatal sepsis have documented rates as high as 170 cases per 1000 live births.[17]

COSTS ASSOCIATED WITH SEPSIS AND ITS MANAGEMENT
Cost Sources

Basic economic concepts and the economics and costs of critical care medicine as a whole are covered in depth in the articles by John Rizzo, Steven Pastores, and John Rapoport elsewhere in this issue, but it is worth noting that the overall utilization and costs of critical care medicine have grown in recent years. Between 2000 and 2005, the national number of critical care medicine inpatient days grew from 21.0 million to 23.2 million, the cost of each of those days grew from $2698 to $3518, and the overall cost of the delivery of critical care medicine in the United States rose from $56.6 billion to $81.7 billion.[18]

Fixed costs dominate resource consumption in the ICU. Studies examining costs among all ICU patients demonstrate that staffing costs represent between 46.4% and 56.1% of total intensive care costs, the single largest proportion of ICU costs. Patient-variable costs are proportionally smaller: medications, including antibiotics, account for between 15.6% and 21.7% of costs; diagnostic procedures and laboratory tests account for between 17.9% and 20.4% of costs; and invasive procedures, such as mechanical ventilation, account for between 3.0% and 6.6% of costs.[19,20]

At all levels of care, septic patients incur consistently higher daily costs than nonseptic patients.[20] Within an ICU population, treatment costs for septic patients are also considerably higher than for nonseptic patients, an effect that can be explained by the prolonged length of stay required for the treatment of sepsis.[21]

Costs for ICU patients with sepsis exhibit a similar breakdown compared with the overall ICU population, with fixed costs comprising the majority of the total. In a study of septic patients in UK intensive care units, the two most costly expenditures were nursing care and medications. Among patients who were septic on admission, the median daily cost of nursing staffing was $317 (53% of total daily ICU costs), the median daily cost of drugs and fluids was $116 (19%), the median cost of consumables was $83 (14%), and the median cost of medical staffing was $84 (14%).[22] In a study of Swiss ICU patients with severe sepsis, staffing again represented the single largest proportion of costs (51% of total daily costs), followed by medication (19%), laboratory tests (10%), hotel (basic bed) costs (9%), consumables (7%), and microbiology costs (5%).[23]

Because health care systems and infrastructures, along with the pricing and cost of goods and services, vary from country to country, some studies deviate from these general trends. A study of sepsis patients in German ICUs found that the single greatest cost was medication (40% of total costs), followed closely by staffing costs (36%). Laboratory costs comprised 10% of total costs, hotel costs (basic bed costs and nonclinical support services) made up 7% of total costs, microbiology costs comprised 4% of total costs, and disposables represented 3% of total costs.[24]

Because fixed costs such as staffing represent such a large proportion of septic patients' daily costs, length-of-stay (LOS) in the ICU and in the hospital overall represents an especially important contributor to total costs. In a multicenter study examining 1173 episodes of sepsis, Bates and colleagues determined the factors that significantly correlate to longer post-onset LOS and higher total hospital charges in sepsis patients. These factors include admission to an ICU; the use of mechanical ventilation; admission to a surgical service and having had an operative procedure in the operating room; liver, heart, or lung transplant; burn; multiple trauma; bowel perforation or severe pancreatitis; cardiopulmonary resuscitation; acute respiratory distress syndrome (ARDS); cardiogenic shock; total parenteral nutrition (TPN, with or without intralipid therapy); steroid therapy; and a blood culture positive for gram-negative rods.[25]

Costs of Sepsis In the United States

The total annual cost for the hospitalization of patients with severe sepsis in the United States has been estimated at $16.7 billion, and the authors surmise that this figure has probably risen since these data were published.[6] Recent analysis of data from the National Inpatient Sample indicates that septicemia is one of five conditions that accounts for the most expensive hospital stays nationally.[26] Individual episodes of sepsis have historically been costly because many septic patients represent economic outliers, consuming significantly greater than average resources per hospital episode. Like all health care costs in the US, costs of sepsis have risen substantially over the years. In 1978, the estimated excess cost of a case of bacteremia was $3600.[27] More recently, Bates and colleagues examined excess resource use among patients with sepsis in eight academic medical centers. The mean length of hospital stay was increased by 20.5 days in patients with sepsis (27.7 days vs 7.2 days for patients without sepsis). The mean cost of care for a patient with sepsis was $86,231 higher than the mean cost of all other admissions ($103,529 vs $17,298).[25] Another study estimated a per-case cost for hospitalizations due to severe sepsis in the United States at $22,100, rising to $29,990 for patients with an ICU stay and $30,800 for surgical patients.[6] Average costs rose from $19,500 for patients with acute dysfunction in one organ system to $32,800 for patients with dysfunction in four or more systems.

Costs for hospitalization due to severe sepsis decline with age. Hospitalization of an infant is the most expensive, at a mean cost of $54,300. Episodes of severe sepsis incur an average cost of $28,000 for patients aged 1 to 19 years, between $21,000 and $25,000 for adults, and $14,600 for patients aged 85 years or older. Despite the lower cost per patient of treating severe sepsis in older patients, a larger epidemiologic burden among that population means that the national cost for treating the elderly is actually very high. More than half of severe sepsis cases occur among patients 65 years of age or older, and costs for treating these patients account for 52.3% of total national costs.[28]

A study of severe sepsis in a managed care cohort produced comparable numbers and similar trends. The mean cost of a severe sepsis hospitalization was $26,820, rising to $36,218 in patients requiring an ICU stay and $38,036 in surgical patients. Hospitalization costs again declined with age; patients younger than 18 years of age cost the most ($56,629) whereas patients 80 years old and older incurred the lowest costs ($4574).[29]

Costs of treating sepsis may vary greatly by institution. Angus and colleagues noted both increased cost of care and increased length of stay at teaching institutions in comparison to non-teaching institutions.[6] An analysis of resource use in the management of severe sepsis at eight academic medical centers found a wide variation in cost. Mean total charges ranged from $69,429 to $237,898 across the eight centers, potentially partially explained by a variation in post-onset LOS from 15.9 to 24.2 days.[30]

As with any health care intervention, the use of vast resources to treat patients does not necessarily produce better outcomes in sepsis. An analysis of more than 166,000 patients with sepsis at 309 hospitals found wide variation in mortality and cost. One third of hospitals exceeded expected costs of care by at least 10%. No significant association existed between hospital spending and mortality. More hospitals had higher-than-expected costs and higher-than-expected mortality rates (10% of hospitals) than had lower-than-expected costs and mortality rates (7% of hospitals).[31] These and other disparities highlight the need for a comprehensive, quantitative assessment of value, in terms of cost-effectiveness, cost-utility, and related metrics, the paucity of which is discussed relative to sepsis later in this article.

In addition to the large national burden of sepsis care, treatment of septic patients often represents a significant financial liability for hospitals in the United States. Ernst and colleagues' evaluation of Medicare data found that many more patients with severe sepsis, in comparison to ICU patients with other morbidities, incurred costs above the fixed-loss threshold set by the Centers for Medicare and Medicaid Services (23.2% vs 7.2%). Although some cases qualified for outlier payments, hospitals on average recovered only 85.2% of costs in cases of severe sepsis. Among patients with a diagnosis of septicemia, the average loss per case of severe sepsis was $5944, in comparison to a loss of $3093 for non-severe-sepsis ICU patients.[32]

Costs of Sepsis Internationally

The economic burden of sepsis is not a concern unique to the United States and has been a topic of investigation in many countries. **Table 1** demonstrates the wide variability that exists in costs per episode of sepsis. Differences in costs between countries are attributable to differing standards of care, treatment and labor costs, and health care infrastructures. Differences in costs between studies within a given country may also be attributable to differences in study design and other methodological factors.

References	Country	Year	Sepsis Category	Mean Length of Stay (days)	Mean Cost per Episode
Table 1 Country-specific costs of sepsis					
Rosenthal et al[33]	Argentina	2003	BSI	11.9[a]	$4888[d]
Pirson et al[34]	Belgium	2005	Bacteremia	34.6	€18,288
Pirson et al[35]	Belgium	2008	Bacteremia	38.9	€23,548
Vrijens et al[36]	Belgium	2010	BSI	9.9[a]	€4900[d]
Sogayar et al[37]	Brazil	2008	Sepsis	10[b,c]	$9632[e,f]
Letarte et al[38]	Canada	2002	Severe sepsis	10.8	$11,474
Cheng et al[11]	China	2007	Severe sepsis	22	$11,390
Brun-Buisson et al[39]	France	2003	Sepsis	37	€26,256
			Severe sepsis	43	€35,185
			Septic shock	34	€27,083
Moerer et al[24]	Germany	2002	Severe sepsis	16.6[b]	€23,297
Kothari et al[40]	India	2009	Bacteremia	33.2	$14,818[d]
Higuera et al[41]	Mexico	2007	BSI	6.1[a]	$11,591[d]
Flaatten et al[42]	Norway	2003	Severe sepsis		€35,906
Schmid et al[23]	Switzerland	2004	Severe sepsis	12.9[b]	CHF 41,790
Edbrooke et al[22]	United Kingdom	1999	Sepsis		$10,623[f]
Angus et al[6]	United States	2001	Severe sepsis	19.6	$22,100
Bates et al[25]	United States	2003	Sepsis	27.7	$103,529
Braun et al[29]	United States	2004	Severe sepsis	16	$26,820

BSI, bloodstream infection.
[a] Excess length of stay.
[b] ICU length of stay.
[c] Median length of stay.
[d] Excess cost per episode.
[e] ICU cost per episode.
[f] Median cost per episode.

Costs of Nosocomial Sepsis

Health care–acquired infections consume substantial resources, and bloodstream infections (BSIs) constitute a considerable proportion of those infections. An examination of 60,000 discharges in 166 hospitals found that sepsis was the most common health care–acquired complication (infectious or otherwise) in patients having either one or two health care–acquired complications.[43] BSIs are estimated to account for 19% of hospital-acquired infections in medical ICUs, 14% in combined medical–surgical ICUs, and 17% in coronary care units; in each case, approximately 90% of nosocomial BSIs are associated with central lines.[44–46]

A nationwide surveillance study in the United States of more than 24,000 BSIs found that 51% of hospital-acquired BSIs occurred in the ICU.[47] A multicenter study examining patients admitted to 28 ICUs in Europe, Canada, and Israel found that the overall incidence of infection among patients was 21.1%. The incidence of hospital-acquired infections (9.2%) was nearly as high as the incidence of community-acquired infections (11.9%). Extrapolating from data of Alberti and colleagues, 41% of sepsis cases were community-acquired, 26% were hospital-acquired (already infected by ICU admission), and 33% were ICU-acquired among patients staying in the ICU for greater than 24 hours. For patients with severe sepsis, the proportion of cases that were community-acquired dropped to 32%, while 68% were either hospital- or ICU-acquired.[48]

The impact of hospital-acquired episodes of sepsis is of particular concern. As a potentially-preventable phenomenon, nosocomially-acquired sepsis has obvious ethical, clinical, and public health ramifications in addition to significant economic costs. Efforts to control hospital-acquired infections may be not only clinically beneficial but also cost-effective or even cost-saving, even if they require significant up-front investments.

Bates and colleagues found that episodes of nosocomial sepsis were more expensive to treat than community-acquired sepsis cases ($73,212 vs $16,130). However, the difference was no longer significant when pre-onset LOS, or the time in the hospital before the diagnosis or recognition of sepsis, was adjusted for.[25]

An analysis of 550,000 cases of nosocomial sepsis found that the mean attributable cost per episode is far higher in surgical patients ($32,900) than in nonsurgical patients ($5800–$12,700).[49] A study of the costs of antimicrobial treatment in nosocomial BSIs found that catheter-related BSIs incurred the highest mean daily antimicrobial costs (€122.73) of infections with a known focus, followed by pulmonary (€112.80), abdominal, (€98.00), wound (€89.21), and urinary tract (€87.85) foci.[50]

As of 2008, Medicare no longer reimburses for a group of eight hospital-acquired complications, one of which is vascular catheter–associated infection.[51] As other payers follow suit and align financial disincentives with preventable complications—and as the list of nonreimbursable complications grows to include a broader range of BSIs—absorbing the costs of nosocomial sepsis will become a significant financial burden for hospitals.

Intrapathogenic Variation in Costs

Several studies have compared the variation in costs between episodes of sepsis caused by different infectious pathogens. An examination of daily antimicrobial costs in nosocomial bloodstream infections found wide variation based on the causative organism. Antimicrobial treatment of bloodstream infection by *Candida* species was the most expensive, with daily treatment of candidemia costing twice as much as bacteremia (mean €208.01 vs €101.05). Among bacteria, the daily cost to treat gram-positive organisms (€112.33) was higher than the daily cost to treat gram-negative organisms (€84.30). Multidrug resistance increases antimicrobial treatment costs by 50% (€165.09 vs €82.67).[50]

In the largest survey of nosocomial BSIs in the United States, *Candida* spp. were found to be the fourth most common causative pathogen in all hospital patients and third most common cause in ICU patients (9.0% and 10.1% of BSIs, respectively).[47,52] Episodes of candidemia are more expensive than bacteremia, incurring significantly higher mean hospital costs ($30,219 for *Candida* spp. vs $12,305–$21,678 [depending on bacterial pathogen]) and higher attributable costs ($12,617 vs $3693–$6871).[53] Although a growing proportion of candidemia is caused by fluconazole-resistant strains, decreased azole susceptibility was not found to significantly increase hospital charges in candidemia patients.[54]

Staphylococcus aureus is the second most common causative pathogen in nosocomial BSIs, and methicillin-resistant strains account for a growing proportion of infections.[47] Studies of patients with methicillin-resistant *Staphylococcus aureus* (MRSA) bacteremia have found significantly higher costs of hospitalization compared with those infected by methicillin-sensitive strains (MSSA).[55–58] However, patients with nosocomial bacteremias caused by MRSA experience more complicated hospital course before the onset of the infection.[59] Therefore, hospital costs before the onset of the infection may be higher in MRSA BSI patients compared with MSSA BSI patients. In addition, postinfection hospital costs are significantly higher in MRSA BSI patients compared with MSSA BSI patients ($51,492 vs $17,603).[60]

As the third most common cause of nosocomial BSIs, Enterococci are responsible for approximately one-tenth of all cases.[47] A growing proportion of *Enterococcus* infections in hospitals are caused by vancomycin-resistant strains.[61] Hospitalization costs in vancomycin-resistant *Enterococcus* (VRE) BSI patients have been found to be significantly higher than for those with vancomycin-sensitive (VSE) *Enterococcus* BSI,[62] and the per-episode cost attributable to vancomycin resistance has been estimated at $1713.[63]

Costs of the Burden of Illness

Although the in-hospital costs of sepsis are great, patient care costs after an acute episode may be even greater. Weycker and colleagues estimated medical care charges for a cohort of severe sepsis patients annually for 5 years after an index admission for sepsis, taking into consideration all inpatient and outpatient medical and pharmaceutical charges. The mean cost of the index admission was $44,600. By 180 days after the index admission, mean cumulative total medical charges were $68,300. At 1 year, 3 years, and 5 years, the mean cumulative total medical charges were $78,500, $103,600, and $118,800, respectively.[64]

A study tracking postdischarge costs of medical care in a Canadian cohort of severe sepsis survivors estimated that total medical care costs in the first year were CAN$20,859 and in the third year were CAN$7099. In the first year, 88% of costs were due to hospitalization, 1% were due to emergency department visits and day surgery, and 10% were due to physician claims. In the third year, 77% of costs were due to hospitalization, 3% were due to emergency department visits and day surgery, and 20% were due to physician claims.[65]

The costs of sepsis borne by society go beyond medical care charges; human capital and productivity are lost, too. Several studies estimate that these indirect costs (in the form of productivity loss due to work absenteeism, early retirement, or premature death) outweigh the costs of direct medical costs. In studies of the burden of illness imposed by severe sepsis in Switzerland and Germany, Schmid and colleagues calculated that indirect costs to society represent approximately 70% of total costs due to sepsis, while direct medical costs account for only 30% of total costs.[23,66]

COST-EFFECTIVENESS ANALYSES IN SEPSIS

Physician and health economist William Kissick has described the fundamental dilemma of medicine as being between the demand of infinite need for medical care and the availability of finite resources.[67] This dilemma is witnessed acutely in the setting of critical care, where demand for costly interventions is high. As the epidemiologic burden of sepsis continues to grow, cost containment will be crucial to the financial sustainability of critical care units. Consequently, assessment of the joint economic and clinical impact, or cost-effectiveness analyses, of sepsis treatment and interventions will be increasingly vital.

Economic evaluation of critical care can be an ethically difficult subject because forgoing costly and aggressive interventions may lead to loss of life or quality of life within a very short timeframe. This narrow window makes clear the direct consequences of cost saving in ways that are not always clear in the ambulatory setting.

Nevertheless, infinite expenditure is not feasible, and certain interventions may be exceedingly expensive while providing minimal health gains. Cost-effectiveness is an important guiding principle for decision making surrounding the allocation of scarce health care resources.[68,69]

Although many methods of analysis may be used to assess economic impact and value, two approaches in particular are commonly used for economic analysis in health care: cost-effectiveness and cost-utility analyses.[68,69] Cost-effectiveness analysis (CEA) compares the expected benefit of an intervention with its net cost. This relationship is expressed in terms of an incremental cost-effectiveness ratio, in which the incremental cost of the treatment being evaluated (relative to standard care) is divided by its incremental benefit (also compared with standard care). Most commonly, the clinical benefit is measured by the number of years of life saved. A clear weakness of this approach is that not all years of life saved are of equal value. An attempt to overcome this weakness can be made by using cost-utility analysis. This is a type of CEA that examines costs and effectiveness using the quality-adjusted life year (QALY) as the unit of effectiveness. Quality of life is measured in utilities, which are preferences (or values) for health states. The number of life-years saved is multiplied by the utility of the health state to produce the QALY.

Ideally, all health care interventions would be assessed by the methods of CEA, and these analyses are indeed common in many areas of medicine. Until recently, however, critical care as a field has not been as rigorous in making these assessments. When such analyses have been performed, they have usually involved expensive or controversial aspects of care. Within the field of sepsis management, cost-effectiveness analyses have largely concentrated on three areas: measures to prevent nosocomial infections, the use of activated protein C (APC), and the use of integrated sepsis protocols, each of which is discussed in detail in the text that follows.

Nosocomial Sepsis Prevention Strategies

As potentially preventable cases, hospital-acquired episodes of sepsis are a target of much investigation. As stated earlier, 9 of every 10 episodes of nosocomial sepsis are associated with central lines, so prevention of catheter-related bloodstream infection (CRBSI) is an especially active research area. As insurers follow Medicare's lead and discontinue reimbursement for treatment of CRBSI, costs shift from payers to hospitals and effective prevention of episodes becomes financially vital.

Strategies for preventing CRBSIs include proper hand hygiene for health care practitioners, the use of maximum sterile barrier precautions for central venous catheter insertions, skin antisepsis at the catheter insertion site, removal of the catheter as soon as it is no longer required, and routine replacement of intravenous tubing and administration sets.[70] At one academic medical center, the implementation of a standardized training course on maximum sterile barrier precautions for residents and medical students resulted in a 28% decrease over 18 months in the number of catheter-related infections and estimated cost savings of $63,000 to $800,000.[71] At another center, modification of central venous catheter kits to replace povidone-iodine with chlorhexidine gluconate and to include larger sterile drapes led to a decrease in CRBSIs that was estimated to save the hospital approximately $350,000 per year.[72]

In recent years, more enhanced antimicrobial strategies have been investigated for efficacy, including chlorhexidine-impregnated sponges, antimicrobial-coated catheters, and antimicrobial locks (the filling of a catheter lumen with an antibiotic-containing solution that is allowed to dwell to eradicate microbes). Formal cost-effectiveness studies have focused on antimicrobial-coated catheters, routinely finding that such catheters are, in fact, cost-effective through a decrease in the incidence of CRBSIs.

In a simulation by Veenstra and colleagues, the use of chlorhexidine-silver sulfadiazine–impregnated catheter compared with an uncoated catheter resulted in expected savings of $196 per catheter, through a relative decrease of 42% in the level of CRBSI. The cost-effectiveness of these catheters held for as long as an episode of CRBSI cost more than $687. Calculations of incremental cost-effectiveness ratios in these studies was not possible because the intervention provided both greater efficacy and lower costs.[73] This example highlights an important point about cost-effectiveness analyses: the difference between cost-effectiveness and cost savings. The incremental cost-effectiveness ratio (ICER) describes the relationship between incremental net cost and incremental benefit for a given intervention. Calculation of an ICER requires that an intervention produce a benefit at the expense of an increase in net cost. If the intervention produces a benefit in the setting of a decrease in net cost (ie, if a cost savings exists), as in the antiseptic-impregnated catheter study, then an ICER cannot be calculated.

A comparison of both chlorhexidine-silver sulfadiazine–coated catheters and rifampin-minocycline–coated catheters against standard catheters found that both antimicrobial catheters produced incremental savings of approximately $9600 per CRBSI averted. For every patient who received an antimicrobial-impregnated catheter, $165 to $278 would be saved.[74] A recent analysis comparing four types of antimicrobial catheters (rifampin and minocycline-coated; silver, platinum, and carbon-impregnated; chlorhexidine and silver sulfadiazine externally coated; and chlorhexidine and silver sulfadiazine internally and externally coated) found that all four simultaneously reduce costs while increasing QALYs compared to standard catheters.[75]

The Institute for Healthcare Improvement 100K Lives Campaign has advocated for a central-line infection prevention bundle comprised of five elements: the use of optimal hand hygiene, maximal sterile barrier precautions for catheter insertion, optimal catheter site selection, chlorhexidine skin antisepsis, and daily evaluation of line necessity.[76] Halton and colleagues evaluated the potential cost-effectiveness of the implementation of this bundle in Australia, incorporating the costs of the five elements as well as costs for monitoring, education, and leadership associated with the bundle. Using a cost-per-QALY cutoff of AUD$64,000, implementation of the central-line infection prevention bundle was cost effective if national implementation costs were less than AUD$4.3 million over 18 months.[77] To our knowledge, a comparable study has not been performed to evaluate the cost-effectiveness of implementation in the United States.

It should be noted that the results of a cost-effectiveness analysis are not necessarily generalizable; they must be interpreted in the context of the local circumstances of the study setting. Consequently, a cost-effectiveness analysis for a given hospital may not be relevant or applicable to another institution. For example, if Hospital A has a low baseline rate of CRBSI while Hospital B has a high baseline rate, then the cost-effectiveness of an intervention targeted at preventing CRBSI will be different in each hospital. Preventing a single episode of CRBSI at Hospital A may cost significantly more than preventing a single episode at Hospital B, since episodes of CRBSI are less frequent at Hospital A than at Hospital B.

Drotrecogin Alfa (Activated)

Low levels of APC, an endogenous fibrinolytic and anti-inflammatory protein, have been found to be associated with poor outcomes in severe sepsis.[78] In 2001, results from the first large, multicenter, randomized, double-blind, placebo-controlled trial of the use of recombinant human APC, or drotrecogin alfa (activated, DAA), in severe sepsis were announced. The relative risk of death was found to be reduced by 19.4% while the absolute reduction in the risk of death was 6.1%.[79] Studies soon followed evaluating the cost-effectiveness of treatment with drotrecogin alfa.

As with any treatment with a proven mortality benefit, a proportion of additional costs associated with the treatment is due to hospitalization costs for the increased number of survivors and their long-term health care costs. Drotrecogin alfa increases risk of severe bleeding episodes, and therefore brings with it the additional costs associated with those episodes.[80] The majority of costs associated with drotrecogin alfa treatment, however, are drug-acquisition costs.[28] In one American study, the acquisition costs of DAA averaged $7312 per course of therapy, accounting for 9% of total hospitalization costs.[81] Total costs of hospital care for those patients exceeded reimbursement by an average of $18,227.

In the United States, estimates of the incremental cost per severe sepsis patient treated with drotrecogin alfa vary from approximately $6200 to $15,200 depending on the patient population (**Table 2**). The incremental cost-effectiveness of DAA varies widely depending on the severity of sepsis, as evidenced by the range of incremental cost-effectiveness ratios in studies that stratify based on organ failure or Acute Physiology and Chronic Health Evaluation II (APACHE II) score.

By generally accepted limits for the cost-effective of interventions (<$50,000–$100,000 per QALY), DAA treatment in patients with less severe sepsis is not cost effective.[82] Patients with less severe sepsis derive a negligible mortality benefit from DAA[83] while incurring substantially higher costs of care. Fowler and colleagues calculated that whereas DAA treatment in patients with APACHE II scores of 25 or higher cost only $13,493 per QALY gained, treatment cost $403,000 per QALY gained in patients with an APACHE II scores of 24 or lower.[82] Another study estimated an even larger difference ($32,872 vs $958,423 per QALY gained) between patients with APACHE II scores of 25 or greater and those with scores of 24 or lower.[84]

Table 2 shows the results of cost-effectiveness analyses for the use of drotrecogin alfa in severe sepsis in six countries. The variation in results demonstrates the importance of performing country-specific analyses, since clinical practice patterns, patient characteristics, relative prices, availability of alternative treatments, and societal perspectives on acceptable costs vary from country to country.[85]

Ultimately, the question of the cost-effectiveness of drotrecogin alfa may be purely academic since, as with any other intervention, it depends on proof of clinical efficacy. A recent Cochrane meta-analysis assessing the effects of DAA for severe sepsis found no significant reduction in the risk of death but a significant increase in risk of bleeding.[91] An ongoing multinational, randomized controlled trial (PROWESS-SHOCK) is designed to lay to rest lingering uncertainty over the clinical benefit and cost-effectiveness of this therapy.[92] Should DAA be found not to offer any mortality benefit, it cannot be cost-effective.

Integrated Sepsis Protocols

Evidence-based sepsis protocols have the potential to lower mortality but may increase costs by prolonging length of stay and increasing costs of therapy. We have previously reported on the cost-effectiveness of the implementation of the Multiple

Table 2
Cost-effectiveness analyses of the use of drotrecogin alfa by country

References	Country	Year	Patient Group	Comparator	Incremental Cost per Patient Treated	Cost/ QALY	Cost/LY
Manns et al[84]	Canada	2002	All	Conventional care		$46,560	$27,936
			APACHE II ≤24			$958,423	$575,054
			APACHE II ≥25			$32,872	$19,723
			Age <40 yr			$51,930	$31,158
			Age 40–59 yr			$43,319	$25,991
			Age 60–79 yr			$45,652	$27,392
			Age ≥80 yr			$53,989	$32,393
Riou Franca et al[86]	France	2006	All	Conventional care	$7545	$19,686	$11,812
			Fewer than two organ supports		$7400	$29,507	$17,704
			Two organ supports		$7333	$21,570	$12,942
			Three organ supports		$8187	$13,122	$7,873
Dhainaut et al[87]	France	2007	Two or more organ system failures	Conventional care		€ 33,797	€ 20,278
Neilson et al[88]	Germany	2003	All	Placebo and best usual care			€ 14,119
Hjelmgren et al[85]	Sweden	2005	All	Conventional care	€9701	€ 26,232	€ 18,126
			Multiple organ dysfunction		€11,591	€35,124	€24,400

Study	Country	Year	Category	Comparison group			
Davies et al[89]	United Kingdom (using PROWESS data)	2005	Two or fewer organ system failures	Placebo and best usual care	£5139	£6679	£4608
Davies et al[89]	United Kingdom (using EVBI data)	2005	Two or more organ system failures	Placebo and best usual care	£5386	£11051	£7625
Green et al[80]	United Kingdom	2006	All	Conventional care	£6288	£9161	£5495
			Multiple organ dysfunction		£6661	£8228	£4931
Angus et al[28]	United States	2003	All	Placebo and best usual care	$9800	$48,800	$33,300
			APACHE II ≥25			$27,400	
			Presence of shock			$33,700	
Betancourt et al[190]	United States	2003	One or more organ system failure	Conventional care	$6246		
			Two or more organ system failures		$6246		
			Three or more organ system failures		$6262		
			Four or more organ system failures		$6240		
Fowler et al[82]	United States	2003	All	Placebo and best usual care	$10,745	$20,047	
			APACHE II <25		$6851	$403,000	
			APACHE II ≥25		$15,166	$13,493	

Urgent Sepsis Therapies protocol,[93] the components of which are similar to those in the Surviving Sepsis bundle.[94] Implementation of the integrated sepsis protocol resulted in a mean increase in cost of $8807 per patient, which was largely driven by an increased LOS. The bundle was associated with an incremental cost of $11,274 per life-year saved and a cost of $16,309 per QALY gained.[93] Suarez and colleagues analyzed the cost of implementing the Surviving Sepsis bundle in 59 ICUs in Spain and found an increased cost per patient of €1736, largely due to increased LOS, and an incremental cost of €4435 per life-year gained.[95]

Several studies have evaluated the cost-effectiveness of early goal-directed therapy (EGDT) guidelines for severe sepsis and septic shock. In a simulation of EGDT implementation in an ICU, Huang and coworkers found that startup costs to institute an EGDT program were ultimately offset by decreased LOS such that net hospital costs fell by $8978 per patient. Implementation of EGDT increased lifetime costs through greater survival and subsequent post-hospital costs, resulting in a cost of $2749 per QALY gained.[96] A subsequent trial of EGDT implementation in the setting of an emergency department found that LOS was increased, rather than decreased as in the simulation, resulting in a mean increase in hospital costs of $7028 and an incremental cost-effectiveness ratio of $5397 per QALY gained.[97] The authors attributed the difference between their results and those from the earlier simulation both to the assumptions relied upon in the simulation and to the unrepresentative, homogeneous patient population of the simulation.

Unfortunately, implementing sepsis bundles with proven mortality benefits may not be financially feasible in low- and middle-income countries. Research on the implementation of sepsis bundles in developing countries is scarce, but one such study in Mongolia found that only one hospital had implemented any of the Surviving Sepsis Campaign guidelines.[98] Given the absence of even elementary supportive measures in certain settings, some have advocated for the development of alternative sepsis bundles that employ inexpensive but cost-effective interventions.[99–101]

SUMMARY

The economic burden of sepsis is large and growing. Because sepsis occurs more frequently in older patients, the aging of Western populations will continue to exacerbate this burden. These growing costs of sepsis are an important contributor to national health care expenditures. Increasingly stressed national health care budgets combined with changing economic conditions are leading many countries, including the United States, to reassess their health care funding policies.

In this context, the rational allocation of health care resources becomes increasingly important and opportunities for cost savings will be sought. The high fixed costs of ICU care mean that opportunities for cost savings once a patient is septic are limited. In this situation, prevention of sepsis is the key to cost containment. Because the incidence of hospital-acquired sepsis may be nearly as high as the incidence of community-acquired sepsis, prevention of nosocomial sepsis offers a huge opportunity not only for cost savings but also for patient benefit.

Treatment of patients who have failed preventive measures and developed sepsis will likely involve increasingly-costly drugs and procedures in the future. These interventions must be subject to rigorous cost-effectiveness analyses. Historically, cost-effectiveness analysis has been challenging to carry out in the critically ill patient population, but recent extensive economic analyses of the use of APC and of sepsis bundles offer excellent examples for the future.

REFERENCES

1. Bone RC, Balk RA, Cerra FB, et al. Definitions for sepsis and organ failure and guidelines for the use of innovative therapies in sepsis. The ACCP/SCCM Consensus Conference Committee. American College of Chest Physicians/Society of Critical Care Medicine. Chest 1992;101(6):1644–55.
2. Martin GS, Mannino DM, Eaton S, et al. The epidemiology of sepsis in the United States from 1979 through 2000. N Engl J Med 2003;348(16):1546–54.
3. Martin GS, Mannino DM, Moss M. The effect of age on the development and outcome of adult sepsis. Crit Care Med 2006;34(1):15–21.
4. Mokdad AH, Marks JS, Stroup DF, et al. Actual causes of death in the United States, 2000. JAMA 2004;291(10):1238–45.
5. Melamed A, Sorvillo FJ. The burden of sepsis-associated mortality in the United States from 1999 to 2005: an analysis of multiple-cause-of-death data. Crit Care 2009;13(1):R28.
6. Angus DC, Linde-Zwirble WT, Lidicker J, et al. Epidemiology of severe sepsis in the United States: analysis of incidence, outcome, and associated costs of care. Crit Care Med 2001;29(7):1303–10.
7. Dombrovskiy VY, Martin AA, Sunderram J, et al. Rapid increase in hospitalization and mortality rates for severe sepsis in the United States: a trend analysis from 1993 to 2003. Crit Care Med 2007;35(5):1244–50.
8. Watson RS, Carcillo JA, Linde-Zwirble WT, et al. The epidemiology of severe sepsis in children in the United States. Am J Respir Crit Care Med 2003;167(5):695–701.
9. Padkin A, Goldfrad C, Brady AR, et al. Epidemiology of severe sepsis occurring in the first 24 hrs in intensive care units in England, Wales, and Northern Ireland. Crit Care Med 2003;31(9):2332–38.
10. Andreu Ballester JC, Ballester F, Gonzalez Sanchez A, et al. Epidemiology of sepsis in the Valencian Community (Spain), 1995–2004. Infect Control Hosp Epidemiol 2008;29(7):630–4.
11. Cheng B, Xie G, Yao S, et al. Epidemiology of severe sepsis in critically ill surgical patients in ten university hospitals in China. Crit Care Med 2007;35(11):2538–46.
12. Shen HN, Lu CL, Yang HH. Epidemiologic trend of severe sepsis in Taiwan from 1997 through 2006. Chest 2010;138(2):298–304.
13. Cribbs SK, Martin GS. Going global with sepsis: the need for national registries. Crit Care Med 2009;37(1):338–40.
14. Adhikari NK, Fowler RA, Bhagwanjee S, et al. Critical care and the global burden of critical illness in adults. Lancet 2010;376(9749):1339–46.
15. The global burden of disease: 2004 update. Geneva (Switzerland): Department of Health Statistics and Informatics, World Health Organization; 2008.
16. van Dillen J, Zwart J, Schutte J, et al. Maternal sepsis: epidemiology, etiology and outcome. Curr Opin Infect Dis 2010;23(3):249–54.
17. Thaver D, Zaidi AK. Burden of neonatal infections in developing countries: a review of evidence from community-based studies. Pediatr Infect Dis J 2009;28(1 Suppl): S3–9.
18. Halpern NA, Pastores SM. Critical care medicine in the United States 2000–2005: an analysis of bed numbers, occupancy rates, payer mix, and costs. Crit Care Med 2010;38(1):65–71.
19. McLaughlin AM, Hardt J, Canavan JB, et al. Determining the economic cost of ICU treatment: a prospective "micro-costing" study. Intensive Care Med 2009;35(12): 2135–40.

20. Moerer O, Plock E, Mgbor U, et al. A German national prevalence study on the cost of intensive care: an evaluation from 51 intensive care units. Crit Care 2007;11(3): R69.

21. Burchardi H, Schneider H. Economic aspects of severe sepsis: a review of intensive care unit costs, cost of illness and cost effectiveness of therapy. Pharmacoeconomics 2004;22(12):793-13.

22. Edbrooke DL, Hibbert CL, Kingsley JM, et al. The patient-related costs of care for sepsis patients in a United Kingdom adult general intensive care unit. Crit Care Med 1999;27(9):1760-7.

23. Schmid A, Pugin J, Chevrolet JC, et al. Burden of illness imposed by severe sepsis in Switzerland. Swiss Med Wkly 2004;134(7-8):97-102.

24. Moerer O, Schmid A, Hofmann M, et al. Direct costs of severe sepsis in three German intensive care units based on retrospective electronic patient record analysis of resource use. Intensive Care Med 2002;28(10):1440-6.

25. Bates DW, Yu DT, Black E, et al. Resource utilization among patients with sepsis syndrome. Infect Control Hosp Epidemiol 2003;24(1):62-70.

26. Friedman B, Henke RM, Wier LM. Statistical Brief no. 97: Most expensive hospitalizations, 2008. Rockville (MD): U.S. Agency for Healthcare Research and Quality; October 2010.

27. Spengler RF, Greenough WB 3rd. Hospital costs and mortality attributed to nosocomial bacteremias. JAMA 1978;240(22):2455-8.

28. Angus DC, Linde-Zwirble WT, Clermont G, et al. Cost-effectiveness of drotrecogin alfa (activated) in the treatment of severe sepsis. Crit Care Med 2003;31(1):1-11.

29. Braun L, Riedel AA, Cooper LM. Severe sepsis in managed care: analysis of incidence, one-year mortality, and associated costs of care. J Manag Care Pharm 2004;10(6):521-30.

30. Yu DT, Black E, Sands KE, et al. Severe sepsis: variation in resource and therapeutic modality use among academic centers. Crit Care 2003;7(3):R24-34.

31. Lagu T, Rothberg MB, Nathanson BH, et al. The relationship between hospital spending and mortality in patients with sepsis. Arch Intern Med 2011;171(4):292-9.

32. Ernst FR, Malatestinic WN, Linde-Zwirble WT. Evaluating the clinical and financial impact of severe sepsis with Medicare or other administrative hospital data. Am J Health Syst Pharm 2006;63(6):575-81.

33. Rosenthal VD, Guzman S, Migone O, et al. The attributable cost, length of hospital stay, and mortality of central line-associated bloodstream infection in intensive care departments in Argentina: a prospective, matched analysis. Am J Infect Control 2003;31(8):475-80.

34. Pirson M, Dramaix M, Struelens M, et al. Costs associated with hospital-acquired bacteraemia in a Belgian hospital. J Hosp Infect 2005;59(1):33-40.

35. Pirson M, Leclercq P, Jackson T, et al. Financial consequences of hospital-acquired bacteraemia in three Belgian hospitals in 2003 and 2004. J Hosp Infect 2008;68(1): 9-16.

36. Vrijens F, Hulstaert F, Van de Sande S, et al. Hospital-acquired, laboratory-confirmed bloodstream infections: linking national surveillance data to clinical and financial hospital data to estimate increased length of stay and healthcare costs. J Hosp Infect 2010;75(3):158-62.

37. Sogayar AM, Machado FR, Rea-Neto A, et al. A multicentre, prospective study to evaluate costs of septic patients in Brazilian intensive care units. Pharmacoeconomics 2008;26(5):425-34.

38. Letarte J, Longo CJ, Pelletier J, et al. Patient characteristics and costs of severe sepsis and septic shock in Quebec. J Crit Care 2002;17(1):39-49.

39. Brun-Buisson C, Roudot-Thoraval F, Girou E, et al. The costs of septic syndromes in the intensive care unit and influence of hospital-acquired sepsis. Intensive Care Med 2003;29(9):1464–71.

40. Kothari A, Sagar V, Ahluwalia V, et al. Costs associated with hospital-acquired bacteraemia in an Indian hospital: a case-control study. J Hosp Infect 2009;71(2): 143–8.

41. Higuera F, Rangel-Frausto MS, Rosenthal VD, et al. Attributable cost and length of stay for patients with central venous catheter-associated bloodstream infection in Mexico City intensive care units: a prospective, matched analysis. Infect Control Hosp Epidemiol 2007;28(1):31–5.

42. Flaatten H, Kvale R. Cost of intensive care in a Norwegian university hospital 1997–1999. Crit Care 2003;7(1):72–8.

43. Saleh SS, Callan M, Therriau'lt M, et al. The cost impact of hospital-acquired conditions among critical care patients. Med Care 2010;48(6):518–26.

44. Richards MJ, Edwards JR, Culver DH, et al. Nosocomial infections in medical intensive care units in the United States. National Nosocomial Infections Surveillance System. Crit Care Med 1999;27(5):887–92.

45. Richards MJ, Edwards JR, Culver DH, et al. Nosocomial infections in combined medical-surgical intensive care units in the United States. Infect Control Hosp Epidemiol 2000;21(8):510–5.

46. Richards MJ, Edwards JR, Culver DH, et al. Nosocomial infections in coronary care units in the United States. National Nosocomial Infections Surveillance System. Am J Cardiol 1998;82(6):789–93.

47. Wisplinghoff H, Bischoff T, Tallent SM, et al. Nosocomial bloodstream infections in US hospitals: analysis of 24,179 cases from a prospective nationwide surveillance study. Clin Infect Dis 2004;39(3):309–17.

48. Alberti C, Brun-Buisson C, Burchardi H, et al. Epidemiology of sepsis and infection in ICU patients from an international multicentre cohort study. Intensive Care Med 2002;28(2):108–21.

49. Eber MR, Laxminarayan R, Perencevich EN, et al. Clinical and economic outcomes attributable to health care-associated sepsis and pneumonia. Arch Intern Med 2010;170(4):347–53.

50. Vandijck DM, Depaemelaere M, Labeau SO, et al. Daily cost of antimicrobial therapy in patients with intensive care unit-acquired, laboratory-confirmed bloodstream infection. Int J Antimicrob Agents 2008;31(2):161–5.

51. Medicare program; changes to the hospital inpatient prospective payment systems and fiscal year 2008 rates. Fed Regist 2007;72(162):47129–48175.

52. Morace G, Borghi E. Fungal infections in ICU patients: epidemiology and the role of diagnostics. Minerva Anestesiol 2010;76(11):950–6.

53. Shorr AF, Gupta V, Sun X, et al. Burden of early-onset candidemia: analysis of culture-positive bloodstream infections from a large U.S. database. Crit Care Med 2009;37(9):2519–26 [quiz: 2535].

54. Lee I, Morales KH, Zaoutis TE, et al. Clinical and economic outcomes of decreased fluconazole susceptibility in patients with Candida glabrata bloodstream infections. Am J Infect Control 2010;38(9):740–5.

55. Lodise TP, McKinnon PS. Clinical and economic impact of methicillin resistance in patients with Staphylococcus aureus bacteremia. Diagn Microbiol Infect Dis 2005; 52(2):113–22.

56. McHugh CG, Riley LW. Risk factors and costs associated with methicillin-resistant Staphylococcus aureus bloodstream infections. Infect Control Hosp Epidemiol 2004;25(5):425–30.

57. Greiner W, Rasch A, Kohler D, et al. Clinical outcome and costs of nosocomial and community-acquired *Staphylococcus aureus* bloodstream infection in haemodialysis patients. Clin Microbiol Infect 2007;13(3):264–8.

58. Reed SD, Friedman JY, Engemann JJ, et al. Costs and outcomes among hemodialysis-dependent patients with methicillin-resistant or methicillin-susceptible *Staphylococcus aureus* bacteremia. Infect Control Hosp Epidemiol 2005;26(2):175–83.

59. Romero-Vivas J, Rubio M, Fernandez C, et al. Mortality associated with nosocomial bacteremia due to methicillin-resistant *Staphylococcus aureus*. Clin Infect Dis 1995; 21(6):1417–23.

60. Ben-David D, Novikov I, Mermel LA. Are there differences in hospital cost between patients with nosocomial methicillin-resistant *Staphylococcus aureus* bloodstream infection and those with methicillin-susceptible S. aureus bloodstream infection? Infect Control Hosp Epidemiol 2009;30(5):453–60.

61. National Nosocomial Infections Surveillance (NNIS) System Report. Data summary from January 1992 through June 2004, issued October 2004. Am J Infect Control 2004;32(8):470–85.

62. Stosor V, Peterson LR, Postelnick M, et al. *Enterococcus faecium* bacteremia: does vancomycin resistance make a difference? Arch Intern Med 1998;158(5):522–7.

63. Butler AM, Olsen MA, Merz LR, et al. Attributable costs of enterococcal bloodstream infections in a nonsurgical hospital cohort. Infect Control Hosp Epidemiol 2010; 31(1):28–35.

64. Weycker D, Akhras KS, Edelsberg J, et al. Long-term mortality and medical care charges in patients with severe sepsis. Crit Care Med 2003;31(9):2316–23.

65. Lee H, Doig CJ, Ghali WA, et al. Detailed cost analysis of care for survivors of severe sepsis. Crit Care Med 2004;32(4):981–5.

66. Schmid A, Burchardi H, Clouth J, Schneider H. Burden of illness imposed by severe sepsis in Germany. Eur J Health Econ 2002;3(2):77–82.

67. Kissick WL. Medicine's dilemmas. New Haven (CT): Yale University Press; 1994.

68. Coughlin MT, Angus DC. Economic evaluation of new therapies in critical illness. Crit Care Med 2003;31(1 Suppl):S7–16.

69. Gold M, Siegel J, Russel L, et al, editors. Cost-effectiveness in health and medicine. New York: Oxford University Press; 1996.

70. Edgeworth J. Intravascular catheter infections. J Hosp Infect 2009;73(4):323–30.

71. Sherertz RJ, Ely EW, Westbrook DM, et al. Education of physicians-in-training can decrease the risk for vascular catheter infection. Ann Intern Med 2000;132(8):641–8.

72. Young EM, Commiskey ML, Wilson SJ. Translating evidence into practice to prevent central venous catheter-associated bloodstream infections: a systems-based intervention. Am J Infect Control 2006;34(8):503–6.

73. Veenstra DL, Saint S, Sullivan SD. Cost-effectiveness of antiseptic-impregnated central venous catheters for the prevention of catheter-related bloodstream infection. JAMA 1999;282(6):554–60.

74. Shorr AF, Humphreys CW, Helman DL. New choices for central venous catheters: potential financial implications. Chest 2003;124(1):275–84.

75. Halton KA, Cook DA, Whitby M, et al. Cost effectiveness of antimicrobial catheters in the intensive care unit: addressing uncertainty in the decision. Crit Care 2009;13(2): R35.

76. Berwick DM, Calkins DR, McCannon CJ, et al. The 100,000 lives campaign: setting a goal and a deadline for improving health care quality. JAMA 2006;295(3):324–7.

77. Halton KA, Cook D, Paterson DL, et al. Cost-effectiveness of a central venous catheter care bundle. PLoS One 2010;5(9):e12815

78. Yan SB, Helterbrand JD, Hartman DL, et al. Low levels of protein C are associated with poor outcome in severe sepsis. Chest 2001;120(3):915–22.
79. Bernard GR, Vincent JL, Laterre PF, et al. Efficacy and safety of recombinant human activated protein C for severe sepsis. N Engl J Med 2001;344(10):699–709.
80. Green C, Dinnes J, Takeda AL, et al. Evaluation of the cost-effectiveness of drotrecogin alfa (activated) for the treatment of severe sepsis in the United Kingdom. Int J Technol Assess Health Care 2006;22(1):90–100.
81. Higgins TL, Steingrub JS, Tereso GJ, et al. Drotrecogin alfa (activated) in sepsis: initial experience with patient selection, cost, and clinical outcomes. J Intensive Care Med 2005;20(6):339–45.
82. Fowler RA, Hill-Popper M, Stasinos J, et al. Cost-effectiveness of recombinant human activated protein C and the influence of severity of illness in the treatment of patients with severe sepsis. J Crit Care 2003;18(3):181–91.
83. Abraham E, Laterre PF, Garg R, et al. Drotrecogin alfa (activated) for adults with severe sepsis and a low risk of death. N Engl J Med 2005;353(13):1332–41.
84. Manns BJ, Lee H, Doig CJ, et al. An economic evaluation of activated protein C treatment for severe sepsis. N Engl J Med 2002;347(13):993–1000.
85. Hjelmgren J, Persson U, Tennvall GR. Local treatment pattern versus trial-based data: a cost-effectiveness analysis of drotrecogin alfa (activated) in the treatment of severe sepsis in Sweden. Am J Ther 2005;12(5):425–30.
86. Riou Franca L, Launois R, Le Lay K, et al. Cost-effectiveness of drotrecogin alfa (activated) in the treatment of severe sepsis with multiple organ failure. Int J Technol Assess Health Care 2006;22(1):101–8.
87. Dhainaut JF, Payet S, Vallet B, et al. Cost-effectiveness of activated protein C in real-life clinical practice. Crit Care 2007;11(5):R99.
88. Neilson AR, Burchardi H, Chinn C, et al. Cost-effectiveness of drotrecogin alfa (activated) for the treatment of severe sepsis in Germany. J Crit Care 2003;18(4):217–27.
89. Davies A, Ridley S, Hutton J, et al. Cost effectiveness of drotrecogin alfa (activated) for the treatment of severe sepsis in the United Kingdom. Anaesthesia 2005;60(2):155–62.
90. Betancourt M, McKinnon PS, Massanari RM, et al. An evaluation of the cost effectiveness of drotrecogin alfa (activated) relative to the number of organ system failures. Pharmacoeconomics 2003;21(18):1331–40.
91. Marti-Carvajal AJ, Sola I, Lathyris D, Cardona AF. Human recombinant activated protein C for severe sepsis. Cochrane Database Syst Rev 2011;4:CD004388.
92. Finfer S, Ranieri VM, Thompson BT, et al. Design, conduct, analysis and reporting of a multi-national placebo-controlled trial of activated protein C for persistent septic shock. Intensive Care Med 2008;34(11):1935–47.
93. Talmor D, Greenberg D, Howell MD, et al. The costs and cost-effectiveness of an integrated sepsis treatment protocol. Crit Care Med 2008;36(4):1168–74.
94. Shapiro NI, Howell M, Talmor D. A blueprint for a sepsis protocol. Acad Emerg Med 2005;12(4):352–9.
95. Suarez D, Ferrer R, Artigas A, et al. Cost-effectiveness of the Surviving Sepsis Campaign protocol for severe sepsis: a prospective nation-wide study in Spain. Intensive Care Med 2011;37(3):444–52.
96. Huang DT, Clermont G, Dremsizov TT, et al. Implementation of early goal-directed therapy for severe sepsis and septic shock: a decision analysis. Crit Care Med 2007;35(9):2090–2100.
97. Jones AE, Troyer JL, Kline JA. Cost-effectiveness of an emergency department-based early sepsis resuscitation protocol. Crit Care Med 2011;39(6):1306–12.

98. Bataar O, Lundeg G, Tsenddorj G, et al. Nationwide survey on resource availability for implementing current sepsis guidelines in Mongolia. Bull World Health Organ 2010;88(11):839–46.

99. Becker JU, Theodosis C, Jacob ST, et al. Surviving sepsis in low-income and middle-income countries: new directions for care and research. Lancet Infect Dis 2009;9(9):577–82.

100. Cheng AC, West TE, Limmathurotsakul D, et al. Strategies to reduce mortality from bacterial sepsis in adults in developing countries. PLoS Med 2008;5(8):e175.

101. Cheng AC, West TE, Peacock SJ. Surviving sepsis in developing countries. Crit Care Med 2008;36(8):2487 [author reply: 2487–8].

The Economics of Cardiovascular Disease in the United States

Jie Chen, PhD[a], John A. Rizzo, PhD[b],*

KEYWORDS

- Cardiovascular disease • Cost-effective treatment
- Medical treatment • Surgical treatment • Economic burden

Cardiovascular disease (CVD) is the leading cause of death in the United States, accounting for more than 17% of total health expenditures.[1–5] As such, the clinical and economic implications of this disease are enormous. A variety of medical treatments and technologies have been developed to manage CVD more effectively, improving patient longevity and quality of life. Yet in an increasingly cost-conscious economic environment, it is important to understand not only the effectiveness of these alternative treatments and technologies but also their cost-effectiveness.

This article reviews and summarizes the evidence on the cost-effectiveness of broad treatments for CVD in the United States. More specifically, the authors examine the evidence on surgical versus medical treatments for the management of CVD, contrasting treatments and technologies that are particularly cost-effective versus those whose economic value is less well-established.

This report sheds light on the economic value of treatment alternatives and provides guidance on what treatments confer the greatest net benefit and for whom. Such evidence should prove useful at the patient bedside in helping clinicians to allocate ever-costlier medical treatments and technologies more efficiently and at the macro level in assisting policy makers and third party payers in deciding what treatments to cover.

The remainder of this study is divided into five sections. Section I defines CVD more precisely and reviews epidemiologic data on CVD. Section II reviews the economic burden of CVD in the United States. The cost-effectiveness of alternative medical strategies to treat CVD is examined in Section III. Section IV considers similar

The authors have nothing to disclose.
[a] Department of Political Science, Economics, and Philosophy, City University of New York, College of Staten Island, 2800 Victory Boulevard, Room 2N-226, Staten Island, NY 10314, USA
[b] Department of Economics, Stony Brook University, N-637 Social and Behavioral Sciences Building, Stony Brook, NY 11794, USA
* Corresponding author.
E-mail address: rizzologic@gmail.com

Crit Care Clin 28 (2012) 77–88
doi:10.1016/j.ccc.2011.10.007
0749-0704/12/$ – see front matter © 2012 Elsevier Inc. All rights reserved.

evidence on surgical options, and Section V provides concluding and summary thoughts.

EPIDEMIOLOGY OF CVD
Prevalence

CVD (according to *International Classification of Diseases*, ninth edition [*ICD-9*] codes 390–459 and 745–747, and *ICD* 10th edition [*ICD-10*] codes I00–I99 and Q20–Q28) consists of a number of related, sometimes overlapping conditions. These conditions include hypertension, coronary heart disease (CHD) (myocardial infarction and angina pectoris), heart failure, cerebrovascular disease (stroke), and congenital heart defects.[6] Because of the overlapping nature of these diseases, one cannot add the prevalence of each to obtain an overall prevalence for CVD, but the large numbers of persons affected by these conditions in the United States leaves no doubt as to the extent and seriousness of CVD.

According to recent statistics,[6] approximately 82.6 million American adults, or 1 out of 3, have one or more types of CVD, and almost half of these adults are aged 60 or over. Specifically, among all the cases of CVD, 76.4 million are for high blood pressure, 16.3 million are for CHD, 5.7 million are for heart failure, 7 million are for stroke, and 650,000 to 1.3 million are for congenital cardiovascular defects. These prevalence rates vary by age and race/ethnicity according to the 2009 National Health Interview Survey.[7] Approximately 12% of whites and African Americans have heart disease, followed by Hispanics (9%) and Asians (6%). African Americans have the highest rate of hypertension (32%), followed by whites (23%), Hispanics (22%), and Asians (19%).

Incidence

The incidence rates of CVD differ by age and gender. Evidence from the Framingham Heart Study from 1980 to 2003 reveals that the incidence rate is 3 per 1000 men for the decade from 35 to 44 years of age compared with 74 per 1000 men from 85 to 94 years of age. Women have comparable rates but they occur 10 years later in life.[6,8] A recent report by the American Heart Association (AHA)[6] also notes that "before 75 years of age, a higher proportion of CVD events due to CHD occur in men than in women, and a higher proportion of events due to stroke occur in women than in men." Lloyd-Jones and colleagues[9] found that the lifetime risk for developing CVD is 52% for men and 39% for women, and the overall survival rate is 30 years for men and 36 years for women.

Mortality

Death rates from CVD declined in the United States by 27.8% between 1997 and 2007.[6] Nevertheless, CVD remains the leading cause of death, accounting for one-third (33.6%) of all deaths in the United States in 2007.[6] Approximately 2200 Americans die each day from CVD. Indeed, since 1900, CVD has been the leading cause of death in the United States, with the lone exception of 1918, the year of the flu pandemic. The overall death rate due to CVD was 251.2 in 2007. The death rate was relatively higher for white males (294.0), black males (405.9), and black females (286.1) in comparison with white females (205.1).[6,10]

Risk Factors

Risk factors for CVD include family history, poor diet and lack of exercise, being overweight, abstaining from alcohol consumption, and smoking. The prevalence of

CVD risk factors increases with age.[6,11] Blacks (48.7%) and American Indians (46.7%) have the highest prevalence with two or more risk factors for CVD, whereas Asians (25.9%) have the lowest prevalence. The presence of multiple risk factors for CVD is similar for males (37.8%) and females (36.4%), but multiple risk factors are markedly higher among persons lacking a high school diploma (52.5%) in comparison with college graduates (25.9%). The prevalence of multiple risk factors also varies by state, ranging from a low of 27.0% in Hawaii to 46.2% in Kentucky.[11] The presence of multiple risk factors for CVD is markedly higher for low-income persons and for persons who are unemployed.

Controlling these risk factors remains a critical issue for Americans. For example, recent statistics estimate that approximately 34% of US adults are obese (ie, body mass index ≥ 30 kg/m^2). Data from the 2004 Medical Expenditure Panel Survey (MEPS)[11] reveal that only 34% of those diagnosed with heart disease, stroke, or any other heart-related diseases have healthy weight compared with 39% of those without these diagnoses. In addition, nearly 45% of those with CVD engaged in little or no physical activity, 18% continued to smoke, and nearly all the CVD patients met only three or fewer of the five criteria constituting a healthy diet score.[6]

ECONOMIC BURDEN OF CVD IN THE UNITED STATES
Direct Health Care Costs of CVD

CVD imposes a substantial economic burden on health care systems in the United States in terms of direct costs such as hospitalizations, physician visits, pharmaceuticals, and rehabilitation services and indirect costs associated with mortality or morbidity such as the loss of productivity because of premature mortality or short- or long-term disability.[6]

Using data from multiple sources, the AHA[12] estimated that the annual cost of CVD (including heart disease, stroke, hypertensive heart disease, and heart failure) in the Unites States was $457.4 billion in 2006, of which 64% (approximately $292 billion) were direct costs. Other results using data from the 2003 Hospital Cost and Utilization Project are consistent, showing that the average charges of cardiovascular procedures are the highest among all hospital discharges.[13]

Given the high prevalence of CVD, it is not surprising that the direct costs of hypertension are highest among all CVDs, reaching $185 billion in 1998.[14] A similar result ($177 billion) was found using data from the 1996 MEPS.[15]

However, the calculation of the direct cost of CVD in the United States may vary depending upon the methodology and assumptions, such as the assumption of the prevalence rate for CVD and the statistical methodology used to isolate the effects of CVD on costs. In particular, the estimated effects of CVD on costs may be sensitive to the choice of other control variables included in the cost models, especially comorbidities. Thus, a recent update reduced the total direct health care cost estimates for CVD to $167 billion in 2007.[6] This substantial change reflects updates in assumptions about the ratio of CVD costs to total health care costs and the use of more recent data than previous studies. For the updated estimates, the AHA uses data from the 2007 MEPS,[11] instead of the 1995 National Health Expenditure Accounts used previously. The MEPS is a nationally representative data set of the civilian noninstitutionalized population, and it is administered by the Agency for Healthcare Research and Quality. In particular, MEPS provides information on direct payments for care of a patient with a particular disease during the survey year, and these payments include out-of-pocket payments and third party payments such as private insurance, Medicaid, and Medicare. A more detailed description of the methodology and estimates for the AHA updates is provided by Heidenreich and colleagues.[1]

Indirect Health Care Costs of CVD

Indirect health care costs associated with CVD account for 36% of CVD costs in the United States.[16] The strong majority (75%) of these indirect costs reflect productivity losses due to premature mortality, with the remainder largely reflecting productivity losses due to morbidity.[12]

Based on MEPS 2001 to 2005 data sets, Heidenreich and colleagues[1] calculated that indirect costs for all CVDs will increase from $171.7 billion in 2010 to $275.8 billion in 2030. The investigators calculate two types of indirect costs: (1) lost productivity from morbidity and (2) lost productivity from premature mortality. Morbidity costs represent the value of foregone earnings from lost productivity due to CVD. Morbidity costs include three parts: (1) productivity losses among currently employed individuals (eg, job absenteeism and on-the-job productivity losses), (2) home productivity loss (eg, the loss of productivity of housekeeping services),[17] and (3) productivity losses among individuals who are too sick to be employed.[18]

Heidenreich and colleagues[1] estimated per capita work loss days due to CVD using a negative binomial model in which work loss was estimated as a function of CVD, other comorbid conditions, and sociodemographic variables. Then the total work loss costs were calculated by multiplying per capita work days lost related to CVD to "(1) prevalence of CVD (by age, sex, and race/ethnicity) from MEPS, (2) the probability of employment given CVD (by age, sex, and race/ethnicity) from MEPS, (3) mean per capita daily earnings (by age and sex) from the 2008 Current Population Survey, and (4) Census population projections counts (by age, sex, and race/ethnicity).". Heidenreich and colleagues[1] also provide detailed calculations for other components of indirect costs.

Similarly, Grover and colleagues[19] calculated indirect CVD costs by comparing the productivity of individuals with CVD and those without CVD. Productivity losses were calculated using the employment income losses and loss of housekeeping services. The investigators found that the productivity losses decreased with age for both genders. For example, the average productivity loss for men aged 40 to 49 is $9268, and the loss in productivity decreases by approximately $3000 for every 10 years of age thereafter. Similarly, the average productivity loss for women aged 40 to 49 is $7163, and the loss in productivity declines by approximately $3000 for every decade thereafter.

The 2011 AHA report[6] also notes that current estimates of indirect costs due to CVD measure these costs too narrowly, because some cost components are quite challenging to quantify. In their most recent report, only the lost productivity due to premature mortality is presented ($119.2 billion). Estimates of indirect costs associated with CVD thus remain inconclusive.

Limitations

Each of these studies has some important limitations. Although some studies[20] used nationally representative data sets such as MEPS and the National Health Interview Survey, they may not have controlled for enough patients' demographic or socioeconomic variables that might affect CVD costs. Some studies[21–26] only focus on estimates for particular groups, such as Medicare beneficiaries, private health insurance enrollees, or patients from long-term care facilities. Hence, such studies may not be regarded as nationally representative. Many databases used in these studies are based on patient recall and may be subject to recall bias and measurement error.

Despite these limitations, the evidence consistently suggests that the economic burden of CVD is large, highlighting the need to identify the most cost-effective strategies for managing CVD.

COST-EFFECTIVENESS OF MEDICAL TREATMENTS FOR CVD

A study investigating the decline in deaths in the United States attributable to heart disease from 1980 to 2000 suggests that approximately "47% of the decrease was attributable to increased use of evidence-based medical therapies"[6,27] In this section, the authors present some evidence of the cost-effectiveness of the medical treatments for CVD, focusing mainly on pharmaceutical treatments.

Statins for CHD

The literature consistently shows that statin treatment can reduce CHD, a major component of CVD. However, the cost-effectiveness of statin treatment in the primary prevention of CVD has not been fully established. Franco and colleagues[28] reviewed cost-effectiveness analyses of statins and synthesized cost-effectiveness ratios by risk categories of CHD and age. Their estimates showed values of "$21,571 per life year saved for a 10 year coronary heart disease risk of 20% and $16,862 per life year saved for 10 year risk of 30%." The conclusion of this study is that "statin therapy is cost effective for high levels of risk, but inconsistencies exist at lower levels." The investigators also found that "although the cost effectiveness of statins depends mainly on absolute risk, important heterogeneity remains after adjusting for absolute risk." This heterogeneity might reflect the different methodologies used to estimate cost-effectiveness. The investigators recommend that future economic analyses should be more transparent and consistent to reduce the potential for bias and misinterpretation.

Goldman and colleagues[29] found similar evidence that statins as primary prevention have favorable cost-effectiveness ratios in selected subgroups based on cholesterol levels and other established risk factors. They concluded that "current national recommendations regarding medication for secondary prevention are not as aggressive as our projections would suggest, while recommendations regarding the use of medications for primary prevention should consider the cost of medication as well as the risk factor profile of the individual patient." Johannesson and colleagues[30] examined the cost-effectiveness of simvastatin treatment to lower cholesterol levels in patients with CHD. When the analysis was restricted to direct costs, the investigators found that "the cost of each year of life gained ranged from $3,800 for 70-year-old men with 309 mg of cholesterol per deciliter to $27,400 for 35-year-old women with 213 mg of cholesterol per deciliter." When the investigators included indirect costs, the results "ranged from a savings in the youngest patients to a cost of $13,300 per year of life gained in 70-year-old women with 213 mg of cholesterol per deciliter" in patients with CHD. This study thus concluded that simvastatin therapy is "cost effective among both men and women at the ages and cholesterol levels studied." Prosser and colleagues[31] evaluated how the cost-effectiveness ratios of cholesterol-lowering therapies vary according to different population characteristics and found that cost-effectiveness of treatment varies significantly by age, sex, and risk factors. They found that "primary prevention with a statin may not be cost-effective for younger men and women with few risk factors, given the option of secondary prevention and of primary prevention in older age ranges. Secondary prevention with a statin seems to be cost-effective for all risk subgroups and is cost-saving in some high-risk subgroups." Ashraf and colleagues[32] also showed that the average estimated cost per life-year saved with pravastatin in secondary prevention of coronary artery disease (CAD) ranged from $7124 to $12,665 by patients' risk profiles, and concluded that pravastatin is a favorable treatment compared with other widely accepted medical interventions.

Statins for CVD

Recent studies have shown that treating dyslipidemia among patients with CVD is effective and cost-effective.[29,30,33–39] Many studies have calculated cost-effectiveness ratios under the threshold value of $50,000 per year of life saved in primary prevention among high-risk patients.[33,40–42] However, most of these studies only consider direct cost.

Grover and colleagues[19] examined the cost-effectiveness of lipid level modification with atorvastatin calcium. The benefits were measured by "28% and 38% reductions in total cholesterol and low density lipoprotein cholesterol levels, respectively, and 5.5% increase in high-density lipoprotein cholesterol level." The costs included direct cost, for example, Medicare costs associated with CVD, and the indirect cost, for example, the loss of employment income and the decreased value of housekeeping services due to CVD. The results indicate substantial cost savings (up to $50,000 per year of life saved) and increased life expectancy for most individuals in the atorvastatin cohort. Thus, the investigators concluded that lipid therapy with statins can reduce CVD morbidity and mortality.

Simpson and colleagues[43] examined cardiovascular and economic outcomes after initiation of atorvastatin versus simvastatin in an employed population (1999–2006) stratified by cardiovascular risk. They found that atorvastatin use was associated with a 0.8% lower risk of CV events, $213 higher direct medical costs, $159 lower indirect costs, and $54 higher total costs. The investigators suggested that atorvastatin may not be cost-saving for higher-risk patients from the employer perspective.

Other Drug Treatments for CVD

Gaspoz and colleagues[44] found that both aspirin and clopidogrel could reduce the rate of cardiovascular events among patients with CHD. The investigators estimated the cost-effectiveness of the increased use of aspirin, clopidogrel, or both for secondary prevention in patients with CHD. They found that aspirin for secondary prevention of CHD was more cost-effective than clopidogrel.

Cardiac Rehabilitation

Cardiac rehabilitation is commonly used after myocardial infarction to coordinate exercise training and secondary preventive services. A cost-effectiveness analysis was conducted comparing the relative economic value of cardiac rehabilitation in relation to other common interventions.[45] Cardiac rehabilitation was found to be quite cost-effective, costing $4950 per life year saved in 1995.

Implantable Cardioverter-Defibrillator

The implantable cardioverter-defibrillator (ICD) is an expensive, widely used device for severe ventricular arrhythmias.[46] Kupersmith and colleagues[47] analyzed the cost-effectiveness of ICD compared with electrophysiology-guided drug therapy. The investigators analyzed Michigan Medicare discharge abstracts (1989–1992) and included cost data for physician visits, tests, and ICD charges. The results indicated that ICD cost approximately $31,100 per year of life saved.

Summary

Generally speaking, cost-effectiveness of medical treatments for CVD is heterogeneous. Some studies only calculate direct medical care cost and do not account for indirect costs. Some studies demonstrate cost-effectiveness for particular groups of patients, for example patients from a particular physician clinic. But such evidence may not be generalizable to patients in other settings. Most studies also note that separate cost-effectiveness estimates should be performed for different subgroups of patients, for example those with different risk factors.

The evidence on the cost-effectiveness of medical treatments is fairly consistent, however. A number of studies demonstrate that statins are cost-effective for treating hypertension, as are other drugs such as aspirin. Cardiac rehabilitation, implantable defibrillators, and other devices may also be cost-effective treatments, at least in certain subgroups of patients.

COST-EFFECTIVENESS OF SURGICAL TREATMENTS FOR CVD

A recent report by the AHA notes that approximately 6.8 million inpatient cardiovascular operations or procedures were performed in the United States in 2007.[6] Among these procedures, coronary artery bypass graft (CABG) and percutaneous coronary intervention (PCI) are the most common major procedures performed in the United States.[48,49]

The AHA report further noted that approximately 622,000 patients received PCI in 2007.[6] The mortality rate for PCI has remained stable despite an increase in risk.[50] Moreover, some 232,000 patients underwent a total of 408,000 CABG procedures in 2007. Although these procedures have become increasingly common, risk-adjusted mortality for CABG has declined significantly during the past decade.[6]

PCI Versus CABG

Bravata and colleagues[51] reviewed the comparative effectiveness of PCI and CABG. In particular, they reviewed the evidence from 23 randomized controlled trials, finding that, "Compared with PCI, CABG was more effective in relieving angina and led to fewer repeated revascularizations but had a higher risk for procedural stroke. Survival to 10 years was similar for both procedures."

Another study compared CABG with PCI in high-risk patients with medically refractory ischemia. The study found that PCI was almost 20% cheaper than CABG and just as effective over a 5-year follow-up period.[52] More specifically, the investigators found that total costs for PCI were $63,896 versus $84,364 for CABG patients—a difference of $20,468. The corresponding figures after 5 years were $81,790 for PCI and $100,522 for CABG—a difference of $18,732. Survival was similar in both treatment arms at 3 or 5 years.

Previous studies have demonstrated that, despite higher initial costs, long-term costs with CABG in multivessel CAD are similar to those for PCI. However, the impact of drug-eluting stents on these results is unknown. Cohen and colleagues[53] used the SYNTAX trial, randomizing 1800 patients with left main or three-vessel CAD to either CABG or PCI using paclitaxel-eluting stents. Although PCI cost less, cost-effectiveness varied considerably, depending on the nature and extent of disease. The investigators found that, among patients with three-vessel or left main CAD, PCI is more cost-effective over a 1-year follow-up period for patients with low to moderate angiographic complexity, whereas CABG is preferred for patients with high angiographic complexity. Serruys and colleagues[54] demonstrated that coronary stenting for multivessel disease is less costly than bypass surgery over a 1-year follow-up and offers the same degree of protection against death, stroke, and myocardial infarction. However, stenting is more likely to require repeat revascularization.

In a review of the evidence, Kupersmith and colleagues[47] noted that, "Cost-effectiveness of CABG surgery depends on targeting; eg, it is highly effective for such conditions as left-main and three-vessel disease but not for lesser disease. PCI appears to be cost-effective in situations where there is clinical consensus for its use, eg, severe ischemia and one-vessel disease, but requires further analysis based on randomized data; coronary stents also appear to be cost-effective. Cardiac transplant appears to be cost-effective but requires further study."

In 2006, approximately three-quarters of stents implanted during PCI were drug-eluting stents compared with one-quarter that were bare metal stents (BMS).[6,55] There is only limited evidence on the cost-effectiveness of drug-eluting stents compared with BMS over a time horizon exceeding 1 year. Bischof and colleagues[56] constructed a Markov model using clinical outcomes data from a meta analysis that "included 17 randomized controlled trials comparing drug-eluting versus BMS with a minimum follow-up of 1 year (n = 8,221) and a maximum follow-up of 3 years (n = 4,105) in patients with chronic coronary artery disease." The investigators measured costs as reimbursement rates for diagnosis-related groups from the United States Centers for Medicare and Medicaid Services. Costs and benefits were discounted at 3% annually, and costs were expressed in 2007 US dollars. The investigators found that "drug-eluting stents are not cost-effective compared with BMS when implanted in unselected patients with symptomatic ischemic coronary artery disease." Serruys and colleagues[57] compared PCI and CABG for treating patients with previously untreated three-vessel and/or left main CAD. Consistent with previous research, they found evidence to support CABG as the standard of care for patients with three-vessel or left main CAD, because CABG, compared with PCI, produced lower rates of the combined end point of major adverse cardiac or cerebrovascular events at 1 year in these patients.

Summary

As with medical treatments, there is considerable evidence that surgical options for treating CVD are cost-effective when tailored to the patients' needs and extent of disease. CABG is generally more cost-effective in patients with significant disease, whereas the less costly PCI is generally preferable for patients with less extensive vessel disease. Newer generations of stents are being compared with the standard of care in an effort to demonstrate further opportunities for providing cost-effective care while enhancing patient outcomes.

DISCUSSION

CVD is a leading cause of mortality and morbidity in the United States. It has been estimated that the annual cost of CVD (including heart disease, CHD, stroke, hypertensive heart disease, heart failure) in the United States was $457.4 billion in 2006, of which 64% (approximately $292 billion) were direct costs.[12] The authors' study reviews the evidence on the economic costs of CVD in the United States and the cost-effectiveness of medical and surgical alternatives for managing patients with CVD.

Given rapid advances in technologies, economic and cost-effectiveness analyses are often needed early in conjunction with the research and development phase. Because comprehensive economic analyses, especially those from the societal perspective, often attempt to assess the full economic impact over the course of a patient's and population's lifetime, we therefore depend on simulation models using forecasts of outcomes. One cannot wait 10 years, for example, to evaluate a medical treatment, because by then new treatments are being used. Moreover, outcomes for CVD patients may take a number of years to manifest. Hence, simulation modeling, often involving forecasts of outcomes over multiyear time horizons, is important to fully assess the costs and benefits of medical and surgical treatments for CVD. At the same time, data limitations as well as the interests of various stakeholders may argue for shorter time horizons. Managed care organizations, for example, may be more interested in evaluating CVD treatment and technologies over relatively brief time horizons, given the turnover in their covered populations.

In any event, available evidence on the direct and indirect costs of CVD varies across studies because of differences in assumptions, methodologies, and data sources. However, nearly every study concludes that CVD is one of the most expensive diseases in the United States.

The evidence on cost-effectiveness analysis of medical and surgical treatment of CVD is considerable. Some studies pertain only to particular groups of patients and may not be generalizable. But overall, the evidence on the cost-effectiveness of these treatments is relatively consistent. This consistency is particularly true of the more common, established treatments. Thus, there is considerable evidence that statins are cost-effective treatments for managing hypertension and that CABG and PCI are cost-effective revascularization techniques, especially when given to the most appropriate groups of patients. Nonetheless, the cost-effectiveness of a particular treatment might be substantially different according to different patient population characteristics or risk factors. Some studies have also shown that new treatments involve only marginal clinical gains that may not differ meaningfully from more established treatments.

Some studies have indicated the potential beneficial effects of healthy lifestyle in reducing CVD burdens and improving CVD outcomes and longevity. These studies emphasize that preventing CVD risk factors from developing at younger ages may be the key to successful aging, and they underline the importance of prevention in controlling CVD. In light of this concept, the AHA has expressed its commitment to achieving the following goals: "By 2020, to improve the cardiovascular health of all Americans by 20%, while reducing deaths from cardiovascular disease and stroke by 20%," which encompasses seven health behaviors (lean body mass, avoidance of smoking, participation in physical activity, and healthy dietary intake consistent with a Dietary Approaches to Stop Hypertension-like eating pattern) and health factors (untreated total cholesterol <200 mg/dL, untreated blood pressure <120/<80 mm Hg, and fasting blood glucose <100 mg/dL). "To achieve improvements in cardiovascular health, all segments of the population will need to focus on improved cardiovascular health behaviors, in particular, with regard to diet and weight, as well as on an increase in physical activity and further reduction of the prevalence of smoking." Efforts at prevention through education and other strategies to modify risky behaviors hold great promise, if only compliance can be achieved. However, modifying diet, exercise, and other behaviors is itself challenging, suggesting that medical and surgical treatments will remain key strategies for managing CVD.

REFERENCES

1. Heidenreich P, Trogdon J, Khavjou O, et al. Forecasting the future of cardiovascular disease in the United States: a policy statement from the American Heart Association. Circulation 2011;123:933–44.
2. Trogdon JG, Finkelstein EA, Nwaise IA, et al. The economic burden of chronic cardiovascular disease for major insurers. Health Promot Pract 2007;8:234–42.

3. Lloyd-Jones DM, Hong Y, Labarthe D, et al. Defining and setting national goals for cardiovascular health promotion and disease reduction: The American Heart Association's Strategic Impact Goal through 2020 and beyond. Circulation 2010;121:586–613.

4. Cohen JW, Krauss NA. Spending and service use among people with the fifteen most costly medical conditions, 1997. Health Aff (Millwood) 2003;22:129–38.

5. Russell MW, Huse DM, Drowns S, et al. Direct medical costs of coronary artery disease in the United States. Am J Cardiol 1998;81:1110–5.

6. Roger V, Go A, Lloyd-Jones DM, et al. Heart disease and stroke statistics–2011 update: a report from the American Heart Association. Circulation 2011;123:e18–209.

7. Pleis JR, Ward BW, Lucas JW. Summary health statistics for U.S. adults: National Health Interview Survey, 2009. Vital Health Stat 10. No. 249;2010. Available at: http://www.cdc.gov/nchs/data/series/sr_10/sr10_249.pdf. Accessed September 21, 2011.

8. National Institutes of Health; National Heart, Lung, and Blood Institute. Incidence and prevalence: 2006 chart book on cardiovascular and lung diseases. Bethesda (MD): National Heart, Lung, and Blood Institute; 2006. Available at: http://www.nhlbi.nih.gov/resources/docs/06a_ip_chtbk.pdf. Accessed September 16, 2011.

9. Lloyd-Jones DM, Leip EP, Larson MG, et al. Prediction of lifetime risk for cardiovascular disease by risk factor burden at 50 years of age. Circulation 2006;113:791–8.

10. Sekikawa A, Kuller LH. Striking variation in coronary heart disease mortality in the United States among black and white women aged 45-54 by state. J Womens Health Gend Based Med. 2000;9(5):545–58.

11. Soni A. Personal health behaviors for heart disease prevention among the U.S. adult civilian noninstitutionalized population, 2004. MEPS Statistical Brief No. 165. Rockville (MD): Agency for Healthcare Research and Quality; March 2007. Available at: http://meps.ahrq.gov/mepsweb/data_files/publications/st165/stat165.pdf.   Accessed September 27, 2011.

12. Thom T. et al. Heart disease and stroke statistics—2006 update: a report from the American Heart Association Statistics Committee and Stroke Statistics Subcommittee. Circulation 2006;113(6):e85–151.

13. Mensah G, Brown D. An overview of cardiovascular disease burden in the United States. Health Aff (Millwood) 2007;26(1):38–48.

14. Hodgson TA, Cai L. Medical care expenditures for hypertension, its complications, and its comorbidities. Med Care 2001;39:599–615.

15. Druss BG, Marcus SC, Olfson M, et al. Comparing the national economic burden of five chronic conditions. Health Aff (Millwood) 2001;20:233–41.

16. Tarride J, Lim M, DesMeules M, et al. A review of the cost of cardiovascular disease. Can J Cardiol 2009;25(6):e195–202.

17. Rice DP, Hodgson TA, Kopstein AN. The economic costs of illness: a replication and update. Health Care Financ Rev 1985;7:61–80.

18. Haddix AC, Teutsch SM, Corso PS. Prevention effectiveness: a guide to decision analysis and economic evaluation. 2nd edition. New York: Oxford University Press; 2003.

19. Grover S, Ho V, Lavoie F, et al. The importance of indirect costs in primary cardiovascular disease prevention. Arch Intern Med 2003;163:333–9.

20. Wang G, Pratt M, Macera CA, et al. Physical activity, cardiovascular disease, and medical expenditures in U.S. adults. Ann Behav Med 2004;28:88–94.

21. Samsa GP, Bian J, Lipscomb J, et al. Epidemiology of recurrent cerebral infarction: a Medicare claims-based comparison of first and recurrent strokes on 2-year survival and cost. Stroke 1999;30:338–49.
22. Sloan FA, Taylor DH Jr, Picone G. Costs and outcomes of hip fracture and stroke, 1984 to 1994. Am J Public Health 1999;89:935–7.
23. Amin S, Mullins C, Duncan B, et al. Direct health care costs for treatment of diabetes mellitus and hypertension in an IPA-group-model HMO. Am J Health Syst Pharm 1999;56:1515–20.
24. Garis RI, Farmer KC. Examining costs of chronic conditions in a Medicaid population. Manag Care 2002;11:43–50.
25. Goetzel R, Long S, Ozminkowski R, et al. Health, absence, disability, and presenteeism cost estimates of certain physical and mental health conditions affecting U.S. employers. J Occup Environ Med 2004;46:398–412.
26. Xuan J, Duong PT, Russo PA, et al. The economic burden of congestive heart failure in a managed care population. Am J Manag Care 2000;6:693–700.
27. Ford ES, Ajani UA, Croft JB, et al. Explaining the decrease in U.S. deaths from coronary disease, 1980-2000. N Engl J Med 2007;356:2388–98.
28. Franco O, Peeters A, Looman C, et al. Cost effectiveness of statins in coronary heart disease. J Epidemiol Community Health 2005;59:927–33.
29. Goldman L, Weinstein MC, Goldman PA, et al. Cost-effectiveness of HMG-CoA reductase inhibition for primary and secondary prevention of coronary heart disease. JAMA 1991;265:1145–51.
30. Johannesson M, Jönsson B, Kjekshus J, et al. Cost effectiveness of simvastatin treatment to lower cholesterol levels in patients with coronary heart disease. N Engl J Med 1997;336:332–6
31. Prosser L, Stinnett A, Goldman P, et al. Cost-effectiveness of cholesterol-lowering therapies according to selected patient characteristics. BMJ 1996;312:1443.
32. Ashraf T, Hay J, Pitt B, et al. Cost-effectiveness of pravastatin in secondary prevention of coronary artery disease. Am J Cardiol 1996;78:409–14.
33. Goldman L, Garber AM, Grover SA, et al. 27th Bethesda Conference: matching the intensity of risk factor management with the hazard for coronary disease events. Task Force 6. Cost effectiveness of assessment and management of risk factors. J Am Coll Cardiol 1996;27:1020–30.
34. Downs JR, Clearfield M, Weis S, et al. Primary prevention of acute coronary events with lovastatin in men and women with average cholesterol levels: results of AFCAPS/TexCAPS (Air Force/Texas Coronary Atherosclerosis Prevention Study). JAMA 1998;279:1615–22.
35. Grover SA, Paquet S, Levinton C, et al. Estimating the benefits of modifying risk factors of cardiovascular disease: a comparison of primary vs secondary prevention. Arch Intern Med 1998;158:655–62.
36. Pletcher MJ, Lazar L, Domingo K, et al. Comparing impact and cost-effectiveness of primary prevention strategies for lipid-lowering. Ann Int Med 2009;150(4):243–54.
37. Pharoah P, Hollingworth W. Cost effectiveness of lowering cholesterol concentration with statins in patients with and without pre-existing coronary heart disease: life table method applied to health authority population. BMJ 1996;312(7044):1443–8.
38. Ward S, Lloyd Jones M, Pandor A, et al. A systematic review and economic evaluation of statins for the prevention of coronary events. Health Technol Assess 2007;11(14):1–160.
39. Rich M, Nease R. Cost-effectiveness analysis in clinical practice. The case of health failure. Arch Intern Med 1999;159:1690–700.

40. Hamilton V, Racicot FE, Zowall H, et al. The cost-effectiveness of HMG-CoA reductase inhibitors to prevent coronary heart disease: estimating the benefits of raising HDL-C. JAMA 1995;273:1032–8.

41. Glick H, Heyse JF, Thompson D, et al. A model for evaluating the cost-effectiveness of cholesterol-lowering treatment. Int J Technol Assess Health Care 1992;8:719–34.

42. Kinosian BP, Eisenberg JM. Cutting into cholesterol: cost-effective alternatives for treating hypercholesterolemia. JAMA 1988;259:2249–54.

43. Simpson R, Signorovitch J, Ramakrishnan K, et al. Cardiovascular and economic outcomes after initiation of atorvastatin versus simvastatin in an employed population stratified by cardiovascular risk. Am J Ther 2010. [Epub ahead of print].

44. Gaspoz J, Coxson P, Goldman P, et al. Cost effectiveness of aspirin, clopidogrel, or both for secondary prevention of coronary heart disease. N Engl J Med 2002;346: 1800–6.

45. Ades P, Pashkow F, Nestor J. Cost-effectiveness of cardiac rehabilitation after myocardial infarction. J Cardiopulm Rehabil 1997;17(4):222–31.

46. Sanders GD, Kong MH, Al-Khatib SM, et al. Cost-effectiveness of implantable cardioverter defibrillators in patients >or=65 years of age. Am Heart J 2010;160(1): 122–31.

47. Kupersmith J, Rovner M, Hogan A, et al. Cost-effectiveness analysis in heart disease, part III: ischemia, congestive heart failure, and arrhythmias. Prog Cardiovasc Dis 1995;37(5):307–46.

48. DeFrances CJ, Hall MJ. 2005 National Hospital Discharge Survey. Adv Data 2007:1–19.

49. Singh A. Percutaneous coronary intervention vs coronary artery bypass grafting in the management of chronic stable angina: a critical appraisal. J Cardiovasc Dis Res 2010;1(2):54–8.

50. Holmes JS, Kozak LJ, Owings MF. Use and in-hospital mortality associated with two cardiac procedures, by sex and age: national trends, 1990–2004. Health Aff (Millwood) 2007;26:169–77.

51. Bravata D, Gienger A, McDonald K, et al. Systematic review: the comparative effectiveness of percutaneous coronary intervention and coronary artery bypass graft surgery. Ann Intern Med 2007;147(10):703–16.

52. Stroupe KT, Morrison DA, Hlatky M, et al. Cost-effectiveness of coronary artery bypass grafts versus percutaneous coronary intervention for revascularization of high-risk patients. Circulation 2006;114:1251–7

53. Cohen DJ, Lavelle TA, Hout B, et al. Economic outcomes of percutaneous coronary intervention with drug-eluting stents versus bypass surgery for patients with left main or 3-vessel coronary artery disease: one-year results from the SYNTAX trial. Catheter Cardiovasc Interv 2011.

54. Serruys PW, Unger F, Sousa E, et al. Comparison of coronary-artery bypass surgery and stenting for the treatment of multivessel disease. N Engl J Med 2001;344:1117–24.

55. US Food and Drug Administration, Circulatory System Devices Panel. Meeting minutes, December 8, 2006, Washington, DC. Available at: http://www.fda.gov/ohrms/dockets/ac/06/transcripts/2006-4253t2.rtf. Accessed September 21, 2011.

56. Bischof M, Briel M, Bucher HC, et al. Cost-effectiveness of drug-eluting stents in a US Medicare setting: a cost-utility analysis with 3-year clinical follow-up data. Value Health 2009;12(5):649–56.

57. Serruys PW, Morice MC, Kappetein AP, et al. Percutaneous coronary intervention versus coronary-artery bypass grafting for severe coronary artery disease. N Engl J Med 2009;360(10):961–72.

Economic Aspects of Preventing Health Care–Associated Infections in the Intensive Care Unit

Marya D. Zilberberg, MD, MPH[a,b,c],*Andrew F. Shorr, MD, MPH[d,e]

KEYWORDS

- Ventilator-associated pneumonia
- Health care–associated infections • Cost-effectiveness
- Ventilator-associated pneumonia bundle

In response to the Institute's of Medicine 1999 report "To err is human,"[1] policymakers, payers, and physicians have placed substantial emphasis on the prevention of nosocomial complications. Shocked by the sheer magnitude of preventable morbidity and mortality, a concerted effort has begun to change the way health care is delivered. With renewed vigor, the quality improvement (QI) movement has grown exponentially in recent years, as evidenced by a sharp rise in both research dollars directed at QI and the influence of organizations and initiatives addressing QI. With the knowledge that health care–associated infections (HAIs) occur in an estimated 1.7 million cases annually in the United States, cause 99,000 deaths, and cost between $28 and $33 billion,[2,3] inaction was not an option.

Historically, infectious complications such as ventilator-associated pneumonia (VAP) and catheter-related bloodstream infection (CRBSI) were essentially expected

---

The authors received no funding for the current work. Dr Zilberberg has received research and/or consulting funds from Johnson & Johnson, Astellas Pharma US, Inc., Bard, Forest and Pfizer, and holds stock in Johnson & Johnson. She received research support from the manufacturer to develop the cost-effectiveness model for the silver-coated ETT mentioned in this article. Dr Shorr has served as a consultant, speaker, or investigator for Astellas, Bard, Covidien, Bayer, Esai, Eli Lilly, Forrest, Theravance, and Trius. He received research support from the manufacturers to develop the cost-effectiveness models for both of the endotracheal tubes mentioned in this article.

[a] Department of Biostatistics and Epidemiology, School of Public Health and Health Sciences, University of Massachusetts, Amherst, MA, USA
[b] EviMed Research Group, LLC, PO Box 303, Goshen, MA 01032, USA
[c] Jefferson School of Population Health, Thomas Jefferson University, Philadelphia, PA, USA
[d] Department of Medicine, George Washington University School of Medicine, Washington, DC, USA
[e] Department of Medicine, Washington Hospital Center, Washington, DC, USA
* Corresponding author. EviMed Research Group, LLC, PO Box 303, Goshen, MA 01032.
E-mail address: EviMedgroup@gmail.com

Crit Care Clin 28 (2012) 89–97
doi:10.1016/j.ccc.2011.10.005
0749-0704/12/$ – see front matter © 2012 Elsevier Inc. All rights reserved.

and tolerated adverse events. They were seen as part of the natural history of critical illness. This attitude has shifted under the force and flow of numerous QI initiatives. The underlying message bolstering QI has been one that emphasizes bundles of care that incorporate multiple evidence-based preventive measures. The belief is that by bundling several interventions, each shown to be effective in rigorous studies, one can stem the tide of harm. Because of its face validity, this theory has been accepted broadly and translated into various policies and practices. For example, national payers have eliminated the reimbursement for certain nosocomial complications in attempts to align financial incentives with improved utilization of evidence-based preventive strategies. But despite a decade of expenditures on the implementation of such strategies and an accompanying focus on reducing health care–associated morbidity and mortality, recent investigations have concluded that the "quality chasm" has not narrowed appreciably.[4]

The results of studies assessing QI and prevention have admittedly been somewhat more encouraging in the intensive care unit (ICU) than outside the ICU. Because nosocomial infection can both precipitate and worsen critical illness, intensivists' training in prevention long predates the current QI effort. Thanks to long-standing endeavors by the Centers for Disease Control and Prevention (CDC), the National Hospital Safety Network (NHSN, previously the National Nosocomial Infection Surveillance [NNIS]) has clarified the burden of such commonly occurring HAIs as VAP, catheter-associated urinary tract infections (CAUTIs), CRBSIs, and surgical site infections (SSIs).[5] Thus, through knowing the baseline burden of disease one can better understand where to target the most intensive prevention efforts.

Although unquestionably the right thing to do from a clinical and even an economic standpoint, prevention interventions have nevertheless come under scrutiny, even in the face of data suggestive of success.[6–8] Because each HAI results from a complex interaction between the host, the offending pathogen, and the processes of care, skepticism exists as to whether evidence-based algorithms and bundles can eliminate HAIs altogether. More specifically, a candid discussion is warranted to truly debate whether a "zero incidence" effort represents the appropriate goal. This is a particularly important issue to consider given that the determination of the true burden of many HAIs remains challenging. Specifically, many of the analyses examining this question have multiple definitional issues and methodological limitations. Hence it seems possible that the attributable morbidity and mortality of HAIs may be far lower than previously suggested. This is especially true in terms of the issue of mortality, as it is difficult to assess whether a patients dies with or dies from a HAI. Further, does the apparent reduction in the incidence of HAIs, by itself, constitute a "victory" or, alternatively, does it indicate the effectiveness of a specific prevention paradigm? The definitional confusion surrounding case identification for many nosocomial complications undermines the validity of such assessments. As in the case of VAP, a simple alteration in one's diagnostic approach may dramatically change the estimates of VAP incidence and falsely create an appearance of effectiveness, when in reality this change simply reflects reclassification.[9] Therefore, it is critical to look downstream from the HAI (or its prevention efforts) for clues about the effectiveness of the intervention. In other words, the critical endpoints become not the reduction in the HAI incidence itself, but whether this reduction was accompanied by corresponding decreases in the use of antibiotics, length of stay, mortality, and costs. Without any impact on these clinical endpoints, HAI eradication represents a distinction devoid of a meaningful and measurable difference. With respect to economic concerns, this issue is particularly acute because one cannot adequately assess the value of any preventive strategy if one cannot correctly assess the true costs of the complication under study. As an analogy, many intensivists would not adopt novel, complicated therapeutic interventions without clear and convincing evidence that the intervention actually improved important clinical, rather than surrogate, outcomes. However, when it comes to quality, this logical approach seems to have been disregarded and we, as a profession, seem willing to accept less rigorous data. As such, it seems unclear if we are willing to demand that the science surrounding quality in the ICU be actually quality science.

In the medical and public health realm, a conversation about cost not anchored in a dialogue about clinical effectiveness is meaningless. That is, in the absence of an effect, the discussion of whether an intervention costs a trivial $2 or an exorbitant $2 million will likely be deemed moot, because in each case, each expenditure represents waste, in terms of the inability to "procure" a beneficial outcome. Further, the magnitude of the impact of any intervention has a direct bearing on its value: the greater the positive impact and the lower the cost, the more cost-effective is the intervention. Finally, because our preventive strategies typically consist of bundled interventions, the incremental cost to add each of the components of a bundle needs to be measured against the incremental effectiveness such a change brings, particularly when one hypothesizes that there is a diminishing return in the pursuit of the eradication of HAIs.

Because VAP leads to substantial excess morbidity and costs and because it represents perhaps the most common ICU-acquired HAI, it provides a relevant case study in how to evaluate effectiveness and costs of infection and infection prevention in the ICU. In fact, several features of the literature surrounding VAP and its prevention illustrate some of the potential pitfalls of the QI science. First, VAP definitional issues may have led researchers to overestimate the actual burden of VAP, putting into question whether or not VAP incidence alone is a relevant endpoint. Second, the research into VAP prevention has dramatic limitations, some of which stem from definitional uncertainties, population-specific and geography-specific VAP epidemiology, and the questionable validity of some of the "evidence-based" recommendations. Third, enumeration of the real-world benefits of the accepted VAP prevention paradigms is still lacking or at least severely limited.

VAP

VAP accounts for nearly one third of all HAI and is responsible for more than 50% of all ICU antibiotic utilization.[5] Patient mix has a critical impact on its incidence, with slightly more than 2 cases per 1000 mechanical ventilation (MV) days occurring in medical ICUs and nearly 11 cases per 1000 MV days among burn patients.[10] Geography is another critical factor. An extensive international survey of ICUs in Argentina, Brazil, Colombia, India, Mexico, Morocco, Peru, and Turkey showed that VAP incidence varied between 10 and 53 cases per 1000 MV days.[11] As mentioned previously, the diagnostic approach to VAP is an important determinant of its epidemiology. Not surprisingly, studies that require isolation of an organism as part of the definition of VAP trade off improved diagnostic specificity for diminished sensitivity, and therefore report lower VAP incidence rates than do studies employing only clinical criteria.[9,10] The additional imprecision of the clinical surveillance definition of VAP, with its unacceptably high inter-rater variability, brings some of the reported estimates of the burden of VAP into further question.[12] These variations in VAP incidence are important because they can confound the attempts to assess the value of a prevention strategy. After all, without an accurate assessment of a syndrome's current burden it is not possible to quantify the ensuing changes precisely and accurately.

Given the elusiveness of a clear definition for VAP, one must examine important clinical outcomes downstream from VAP in the context of VAP prevention efforts. Yet choosing such appropriate endpoints may not be straightforward. Although mortality attributable to VAP may be limited,[13] there is no doubt that VAP contributes to the overuse of antibiotics as well as to overall excess resource utilization and hospital costs. It is these costs and the potential impact for improvement in economic efficiency and cost-effectiveness that provide the counterbalancing context for evaluating the investment needed to prevent VAP-associated morbidity.

QI efforts in VAP and other areas appropriately rely on the development of evidence-based practice guidelines (EBPGs). One shortcoming of EBPGs is that they are generally cumbersome and require modification to facilitate adoption at the bedside. The hospital-acquired pneumonia EBPG developed jointly by the American Thoracic Society and the Infectious Diseases Society of America (ATS/IDSA) is no exception, as it includes, for example, 21 separate points of intervention to prevent VAP.[14] They are divided into the following categories: (1) general prophylaxis (n = 2); (2) intubation and mechanical ventilation (n = 9); (3) aspiration, body position, and enteral feeding (n = 2); (4) modulation of colonization: oral antiseptics and antibiotics (n = 5); and (5) stress bleeding prophylaxis, transfusion, and hyperglycemia (n = 3). Each recommendation is based on studies of each maneuver tested as a single intervention.

One should note that the quality of the literature supporting some of the recommendations in the EBPGs appears overstated. Although the Grading of Recommendations Assessment, Development and Evaluation (GRADE) working group was formed to address issues of disproportionate subjectivity in guideline development, the current EBPG did not benefit from its framework.[15] As an example of where the evidence is likely overstated, the VAP EBPG recommends routine elevation of the head of the patient bed. This recommendation derives from one single-center (n = 86; 39 semi-recumbent patients vs 47 supine controls) unblinded, randomized controlled trial among respiratory and medical ICU patients. The study site had a baseline incidence density of microbiologically proven VAP that exceeded 28 cases per 1000 MV days. The study was terminated early for efficacy (which often suggests that the extent of the benefit was overestimated) and has not been repeated.[16] Although the study was important in terms of the questions posed and the sevenfold difference in the odds ratio of VAP between the groups, selection bias, low generalizability, the exceedingly high baseline VAP rate, and the study's early termination all undermine the strength of the conclusions one can draw from the data. Yet, without any suggestion to repeat the experiment, the EBPG suggests that semi-recumbent positioning represents a level I, or strongest, recommendation. From here, this intervention becomes one of the five included in a high-profile MV bundle, informing the emerging policy on quality rating and reimbursement.[17] This example points to a general weakness of the effectiveness data and reveals the need to remain cognizant of the cost trade-offs of any novel, or even broadly accepted, intervention.

In response to the need to balance costs and benefits along with acknowledging uncertainty, a number of studies have examined the cost-effectiveness of some of the tested interventions for VAP prevention, especially those interventions—such as newer endotracheal tubes (ETTs)—that are deemed to be costly. In a study comparing costs and outcomes of managing MV patients with a traditional ETT versus one with continuous subglottic suctioning (CSS), Shorr and O'Malley reported a nearly $5000 savings per one case of VAP prevented, despite a substantially higher acquisition cost for the CSS-ETT.[18] When biasing their model fully against CSS, this marginal cost remained a low $14. Similarly, evaluating a novel silver-coated ETT (Ag-ETT) a study found the intervention to be overall cost saving in preventing VAP in the base case.[19] Varying the inputs that accounted for most of the uncertainty in the model resulted in outcome estimates ranging from savings of $34,000 to an expenditure of $205 to prevent one case of VAP. Another intervention found to be not only cost-effective but also cost saving in preventing VAP is the use of oral decontamination.[20]

All of these cost-effectiveness analyses address the adoption of a single intervention at a time, which is of course necessary to determine the marginal value of the intervention under study. Clinically, though, it makes sense to hypothesize that applying some or all of these recommended maneuvers as part of a prevention "bundle," wherein they are employed concurrently, is more likely to result in a greater magnitude of benefit. In that vein, many studies have examined the effectiveness of a group of preventive strategies in reducing HAIs in general and VAP in particular. Yet few, if any, of these studies examine whether or not preventing HAIs has impacted either antibiotic use or clinical or utilization outcomes. In addition, importantly, few of these bundles have been evaluated systematically with respect to their cost-effectiveness or the marginal cost of preventing one case of an HAI.

One of the best known and most broadly utilized bundles for ventilated patients has stemmed from the "100,000 Lives" campaign of the Institute for Healthcare Improvement (IHI).[17] Although initially aimed at improving the general quality of care for those needing MV, many institutions have adopted this bundle as a VAP preventive strategy. The five interventions that constitute this bundle—semi-recumbent positioning, a daily screen for readiness to wean, daily interruption of sedation, prophylaxis against venous thromboembolism, and prophylaxis against gastrointestinal bleeding—are all supported by high-level evidence.[14] Despite the paucity of evidence for this specific bundle's effectiveness,[21] ICUs that agree to participate in the IHI's program must demonstrate a 95% adherence to each of the components to be considered compliant. More importantly, the aim to reduce VAP using this bundle has been conflated in policy and reimbursement conversations with achieving complete elimination of VAP. At the same time, studies that have examined extended bundled interventions to prevent VAP have met with variable results, further suggesting that the goal of the complete elimination of VAP to a zero incidence rate is unrealistic.[22]

One such study by Bouadma and colleagues examined institution of a multipronged VAP prevention bundle in a large teaching ICU in Paris.[6] They developed their bundle based on an extensive observation period in their ICU and included a rigorous definition for VAP. Although their comprehensive intervention did achieve an impressive reduction in the incidence of VAP from approximately 22 to 13 episodes per 1000 MV days, the authors were unable to come even close to eliminating VAP altogether.

The second key study in the VAP prevention as it relates to bundles represents the efforts of the Michigan statewide Keystone collaborative.[8] The CRBSI prevention bundle study in the same cohort of ICUs successfully reduced CRBSIs by instituting a checklist and implementing a culture of change in these ICUs.[7] In their study of the implementation of the VAP bundle, the investigators noted a reduction in the mean VAP incidence from 6.9 cases at baseline to 2.4 cases per 1000 MV days at 28 to 30 months after the bundle implementation.[8] However, several methodologic issues put these results into question. First, and most importantly, the definition of VAP in this study was that used for surveillance by the CDC, the same one that has been shown by Klompas to have unacceptably high interobserver variability.[12] Second, the study was undertaken in Michigan in response to a detection of higher than expected rates of HAI and of VAP in particular. Such outlier status introduces the possibility that the observed reduction in VAP after the intervention was indeed the result of simple regression to the mean. This also limits the generalizability of the results to states other than Michigan. Third, the study was not blinded and therefore subject to preferential misclassification of VAP in the preimplementation versus the postimplementation periods. Fourth, and also because there was no attempt at blinding, the probability of the Hawthorne effect as the explanation for the VAP reduction detected is substantial. Despite these methodologic shortcomings, no elimination of VAP was achieved. Finally, and illustrating our contention that important clinical endpoints are at times ignored in the QI literature, neither Bouadma[6] nor Berenholtz[8] measured the changes in the sequellae of VAP prevention, such as a reduction in use of antibiotics or in other hospital resource utilization outcomes.

Thus, the paucity of high-quality evidence for the feasibility of eliminating VAP implies that there exists the potential for succumbing to the law of diminishing returns: ever-larger expenditures bringing about ever-diminishing results. Because the ICU, like all components in the health care system, must function under the constraint of increasingly limited resources, attention to competing priorities must be a part of every evaluation effort. Unfortunately, few studies address the value proposition of the VAP prevention bundles. Although not a formal cost-effectiveness evaluation, a study by Lai and colleagues attempted to fill this void by addressing the impact of an intensive surveillance and intervention program targeting VAP on costs and VAP reduction.[23] In this prospective cohort study, the intervention, consisting of elevation of the head of the bed, use of sterile water and replacement of stopcocks with enteral valves for nasogastric feeding tubes, and prolongation of the interval between changing of in-line suction catheters from 24 hours to as needed, were both effective and cost-saving.

One important feature of each of the cost-effectiveness studies discussed so far is that each strategy under study was found to be not just cost-effective but also cost-saving. If true, these studies suggest that future interventions should face a higher threshold for adoption. In other words, because the modalities examined were not only more effective at preventing VAP, but also did so at lower overall cost, it makes little sense, and indeed, may even be considered biased or devoid of equipoise, to compare both costs and effectiveness of other novel interventions to what was the less effective and more expensive control in the aforementioned studies. When one considers how one assesses cost-effectiveness and the algebraic relationship between the differences in costs (numerator) and the differences in the effectiveness (denominator) of the two interventions (eg, bundle implementation vs routine care), the lower the numerator and the higher the denominator, the greater the cost-effectiveness. Thus on this conceptual basis, it is easy to see that selection of the comparator is critical to validity of the results and the overall determination of cost-effectiveness and economic impact.

Note that both strategies presented in the preceding text (ie, the novel ETT technologies and oral decontamination) that are shown to be more effective and less expensive when compared to the traditional ETT, are conspicuously absent from the bundle recommendations.[14] Similarly, their use and implementation varies in studies that have examined the effectiveness of VAP prevention.[6,8] The same can be said for the CRBSI prevention practices as they relate to the use of antiseptic-coated central venous catheters (CVCs). This failure to assess the cost-effectiveness implications of such interventions persists despite studies from national payers. For example, a recent rigorous meta-analysis performed by the health care technology assessment group for the National Health Service in the United Kingdom showed both greater effectiveness and cost-savings with antiseptic-coated catheters.[24] Yet many of the studies of cost-effectiveness in CRBSI prevention do not compare the novel intervention that is the focus of the study against what one might consider to represent the new benchmark. Rather, they compare the novel intervention to a strategy of essentially no preventive intervention, which preferentially inflates the observed effect size of the intervention under study.[25]

A single rigorous study to date that has examined the cost-effectiveness of the common bundled approach to CRBSI prevention in the ICU illustrates these pitfalls eloquently.[26] A thorough review of the current literature by these investigators on outcomes of CRBSI prevention efforts illustrates a dearth of tangible data to help estimate the expenditures needed to implement such bundled interventions as suggested by the IHI and the Keystone project. In fact none of the six publications produced by the Keystone CRBSI prevention project gave a clear picture of the associated resource expenditures. For this reason, the authors had to base their models on best guesses for these expenditures.[26]

The second important gap is that none of the studies of the CRBSI bundle included an investigation of its comparative effectiveness relative to antimicrobial or antiseptic-coated catheters. As discussed at length in the preceding text, benchmarking of the bundle relative to a relevant comparator that is both less effective and more costly than other available interventions will bias both effectiveness and the "value proposition" in favor of the bundle. In fact, the model illustrates this point quite clearly. Namely, if the costs of the bundle implementation are minimal (an admittedly unlikely scenario), it is acceptable for it to reduce the VAP incidence minimally from the baseline seen with conventional management. However, when compared to management with antimicrobial catheters, the bundle has to cut CRBSI rates by 30% to 50%, depending on which type of coated central venous catheter is considered as control, for it to be deemed efficacious.[26] As for cost-effectiveness thresholds, the authors report that the bundle "is cost-effective up to a total nationwide 18 month implementation cost of $4,349,730 when compared only to current practice," and that this threshold diminishes sharply to $1,144,465 when certain coated catheters are considered as controls. This statement is made in the context of the Australian cost-effectiveness limit of $64,000 per one quality-adjusted life year (QALY). In other words, comparing the bundle to a less effective and more costly intervention will result in a higher acceptability threshold for cost-effectiveness (higher costs, lower effectiveness) than if the former is compared to an intervention that is both more effective and less costly.

Despite the lack of studies examining cost-effectiveness of bundled interventions to prevent VAP, many parallels with the CRBSI scenario exist. Given the similarity of organizational efforts needed to implement a VAP bundle on the one hand, and the availability of more effective and less costly intervention for VAP prevention than standard care on the other, one can draw parallels to the CRBSI bundle. In addition, VAP as an entity is arguably also more difficult to diagnose with validity than CRBSI, this feature lending an even greater complexity to deriving the value proposition for any VAP prevention strategies. Nevertheless, the information is urgently needed to build a robust cost-effectiveness model for the VAP bundles, in which both the VAP definition and choice of the comparator intervention will be critical to determining the cost-effectiveness thresholds for these protocols. Further, future cost-effectiveness analyses for VAP as for all HAI prevention need to examine the impact not just on the specific HAI, but also on antibiotic utilization and clinical and economic outcomes. Such close examination of the comparative value of HAI prevention strategies is the only way to arrive at the most sensibly parsimonious path to reducing HAIs, without misappropriating already stretched health care dollars.

SUMMARY

Although it is self-evident that earlier attitudes that did not embrace concepts of HAI prevention are no longer acceptable, it is less clear that current practices are optimally effective for this purpose. Because VAP is the most prevalent HAI in the ICU, it provides a relevant case study for evaluation of the clinical and economic of HAI prevention efforts and the resultant cost-effectiveness ramifications. Although clinicians should strive to minimize the incidence of VAP, the complete elimination of VAP down to an incidence rate of zero for policy and reimbursement threshold is not supported by current available evidence and may be subject to the law of diminishing returns in terms of the requirement for more resources to yield a reduction in VAP at lower and lower incidences. The lack of an agreed upon definition for VAP and high inter-observer variability for the VAP surveillance definition put the validity of the current prevention data in question. This diagnostic uncertainty further argues for examining downstream outcomes of VAP prevention, such as utilization of antibiotics and hospital resources as markers of effectiveness. The highly popular bundled approaches to VAP need to be evaluated in the context of this uncertainty, and the efficiency of their value proposition must include comparators that are known to be most effective and least costly in the prevention of VAP.

REFERENCES

1. Institute of Medicine. To err is human: building a safer health system. Washington, DC: National Academies Press; 1999.
2. Klevens RM, Edwards JR, Richards CL Jr, et al. Estimating health care-associated infections and deaths in U.S. hospitals, 2002. Public Health Rep 2007;122:160–6.
3. Scott RD. The direct medical costs of healthcare-associated infections in U.S. hospitals and the benefits of prevention, 2009. Atlanta (GA): Division of Healthcare Quality Promotion, National Center for Preparedness, Detection, and Control of Infectious Diseases, Coordinating Center for Infectious Diseases, Centers for Disease Control and Prevention; 2009.
4. Landrigan CP, Parry GJ, Bones CB, et al. Temporal trends in rates of patient harm resulting from medical care. N Engl J Med 2010;363:2124–34.
5. Richards MJ, Edwards JR, Culver DH, et al. Nosocomial infections in combined medical-surgical intensive care units in the United States. Infect Control Hosp Epidemiol 2000;21:510–5.
6. Bouadma L, Deslandes E, Lolom I, et al. Long-term impact of a multifaceted prevention program on ventilator-associated pneumonia in a medical intensive care unit. Clin Infect Dis 2010;51:1115–22.
7. Pronovost PJ, Needham DM, Berenholtz S, et al. An intervention to decrease catheter-related bloodstream infections in the ICU. N Engl J Med 2006;355:2725–32.
8. Berenholtz SM, Pham JC, Thompson DA, et al. Collaborative cohort study of an intervention to reduce ventilator-associated pneumonia in the intensive care unit. Infect Control Hosp Epidemiol 2011;32:305–14.
9. Shorr AF, Chan CM, Zilberberg MD. Diagnostics and epidemiology in ventilator-associated pneumonia. Ther Adv Respir Dis 2011. [Epub ahead of print].
10. Edwards JR, Peterson KD, Mu Y, et al. National Healthcare Safety Network (NHSN) report: data summary for 2006 through 2008, issued December 2009. Am J Infect Control 2009;37:783–805.

11. Rosenthal VD, Maki DG, Salomao R, et al; International Nosocomial Infection Control Consortium. Device-associated nosocomial infections in 55 intensive care units of 8 developing countries. Ann Intern Med 2006;145:582–91.

12. Klompas M. Interobserver variability in ventilator-associated pneumonia surveillance. Am J Infect Control 2010;38:237–9.

13. Nguile-Makao M, Zahar JR, Français A, et al. Attributable mortality of ventilator-associated pneumonia: respective impact of main characteristics at ICU admission and VAP onset using conditional logistic regression and multi-state models. Intensive Care Med 2010;36:781–9.

14. Niederman MS, Craven DE, Bonten MJ, et al Guidelines for the management of adults with hospital-acquired, ventilator-associated, and healthcare-associated pneumonia. Am J Respir Crit Care Med 2005;171:388–416.

15. GRADE Working Group. Available at: http://www.gradeworkinggroup.org/intro.htm. Accessed June 30, 2011.

16. Draculovic MB, Torres A, Bauer TT, et al. Supine body position as a risk factor for nosocomial pneumonia in mechanically ventilated patients: a randomised trial. Lancet 1999;354:1851–8.

17. Berwick DM, Calkins DR, McCannon CJ, et al. The 100,000 Lives campaign: setting a goal and a deadline for improving health care quality. JAMA 2006;295:324–7.

18. Shorr AF, O'Malley PG. Continuous subglottic suctioning for the prevention of ventilator-associated pneumonia: potential economic implications. Chest 2001; 119(1):228–35.

19. Shorr AF, Zilberberg MD, Kollef MH. Cost-effectiveness analysis of a silver-coated endotracheal tube to reduce the incidence of ventilator-associated pneumonia. Infect Control Hosp Epidemiol 2009;30:759–63.

20. van Nieuwenhoven CA, Buskens E, Bergmans DC, et al. Oral decontamination is cost-saving in the prevention of ventilator-associated pneumonia in intensive care units. Crit Care Med 2004;32:126–30.

21. Zilberberg MD, Shorr AF, Kollef MH. Implementing quality improvements in the intensive care unit: ventilator bundle as an example. Crit Care Med 2009;37:305–9.

22. Klompas M. Ventilator-associated pneumonia: is zero possible? Clin Infect Dis 2010; 51(10):1123–6.

23. Lai KK, Baker SP, Fontecchio SA. Impact of a program of intensive surveillance and interventions targeting ventilated patients in the reduction of ventilator-associated pneumonia and its cost-effectiveness. Infect Control Hosp Epidemiol 2003;24:859–63.

24. Hockenhull JC, Dwan K, Boland A, et al. The clinical effectiveness and cost-effectiveness of central venous catheters treated with anti-infective agents in preventing bloodstream infections: a systematic review and economic evaluation. Health Technol Assess 2008;12:1–154.

25. Central Line Insertion Practices (CLIP) Adherence Monitoring. Centers for Disease Control and Prevention. Available at: http://www.cdc.gov/nhsn/PDFs/pscManual/5psc_CLIPcurrent.pdf. Accessed June 29, 2011.

26. Halton KA, Cook D, Paterson DL, et al. Cost-effectiveness of a central venous catheter care bundle. PLoS ONE 2010;5(9):e12815.

The Economics of Renal Failure and Kidney Disease in Critically Ill Patients

Amay Parikh, MD, MBA, MS[a],*, Andrew Shaw, MB, FRCA, FCCM[b]

KEYWORDS

- Acute kidney injury • Acute tubular necrosis • Economics
- Cost • Continuous renal replacement therapy
- Slow low-efficiency daily dialysis

The kidney is an organ of opportunity cost in the sense that its function is often sacrificed in exchange for the preservation of function of another organ, organ system, or multiorgan process. This occurs either as a result of a physiologic internal compensatory mechanism or from an iatrogenic insult. Physiologic examples include sepsis, congestive heart failure, and volume depletion, in which the development of acute renal failure (ARF) serves as a signal to the physician, via a reduction in urine output or a rise in serum creatinine, that another process is at play resulting in kidney dysfunction. Physicians weigh risks and make decisions to administer nephrotoxic antibiotics (polymyxin, aminoglycosides) or contrast material, knowing that this may result in kidney dysfunction. Fluid management is especially important in the intensive care unit (ICU), where decisions regarding circulatory support and respiratory compromise must be balanced against one another, often at the expense of kidney function. The ICU setting represents the intersection of multiple organ systems that may result in kidney disease. When the severity of acute kidney injury (AKI) warrants consideration of renal replacement therapy (RRT), multiple modalities such as peritoneal dialysis, intermittent hemodialysis, and continuous RRT are considered. In this article, the economic issues germane to AKI and its treatment in the ICU setting are presented.

ACUTE KIDNEY INJURY

Acute kidney injury (AKI) is a common problem in the acute care setting in general and in critically ill patients in particular. In hospitalized patients, the incidence of AKI ranges from 5% to 7% and appears to be rising.[1–4] In a multinational study of critically ill patients, the prevalence of AKI requiring dialysis was 5.7%, and among these patients, the mortality rate was 60.3%.[5] Patients with AKI also have a higher risk for

[a] Columbia University Medical Center, 630 West 168th Street, New York, NY 10032, USA
[b] Duke University Medical Center, 2301 Erwin Road, Durham, NC 27710, USA
* Corresponding author.
E-mail address: amayparikh@gmail.com

Crit Care Clin 28 (2012) 99–111
doi:10.1016/j.ccc.2011.10.006
0749-0704/12/$ – see front matter © 2012 Elsevier Inc. All rights reserved.

developing other nonrenal comorbidities,[6] and when present in conjunction with other conditions, AKI is itself associated with higher mortality.[7-9]

There are multiple causes of AKI, of which prerenal AKI represents the most common etiology in the ICU. If the systemic cause of prerenal ARF is removed or rapidly corrected, renal function usually improves and returns to near normal levels within a short period of time, usually in a matter of days. Interventions to reverse the cause of prerenal AKI include the administration of fluid therapy, vasopressors, and inotropes; management and control of abdominal perfusion pressure; enhancing cardiac output by diversis; and so forth. Aside from volume depletion, kidney dysfunction may result from systemic factors that decrease glomerular filtration rate (GFR) such as sepsis and septic shock. Other common systemic causes of prerenal AKI include a low cardiac output state (myocardial infarction, tamponade, valvular disease), cardiac surgery, major vascular surgery, trauma with hypovolemia, any cause of shock (anaphylactic, hemorrhagic, hypovolemic), hemodynamic instability in association with surgery, liver failure, increased intra-abdominal pressure, and rhabdomyolysis. The recognition of offending agents or minimizing future administration of nephrotoxic agents is an important step once AKI has been identified.

Septic AKI

AKI secondary to sepsis may be due to different pathophysiologic mechanisms that lead to alterations in renal blood flow.[10,11] Estimates of the incidence of septic AKI range up to 46% of critically ill AKI patients.[12,13] In the report of Bagshaw and colleagues, septic AKI was associated with higher in-hospital case fatality rate compared to nonseptic AKI (70.2 vs 51.8%).[12] In this study, septic AKI patients were noted to have concurrent nonrenal organ dysfunction, a greater need for mechanical ventilation, higher markers of inflammation, and a higher ICU and hospital length of stay.[12] These septic AKI patients were also less likely to have preexisting kidney disease and were more likely to recover to RRT independence by hospital discharge compared to the nonseptic patients. The high hospital mortality for septic AKI patients (70%–75%) underscores the importance of this clinical entity and the need for expeditious recognition and intervention whenever possible.[12,13]

Cardiac Surgery–Associated AKI

AKI is a known complication after cardiac surgery and is associated with an increased rate of death.[14] Of the more than 400,000 coronary artery bypass graft (CABG) procedures performed annually, 5% to 30% of patients will develop AKI.[15,16] Although this clearly demonstrates that AKI is a common complication after cardiac surgery, scenarios identified to distinguish the types of AKI associated with cardiac surgery include acute on chronic cardiac surgery–associated AKI (CSA-AKI), AKI before cardiac surgery, and AKI occurring after cardiac surgery.[17] The rates of RRT use in cardiac surgery range from 0.3% to 1.4%.[18,19] For patients requiring RRT, the mortality rate jumps to 50% to 90%.[20] ICU costs, postoperative costs, and length of stay are higher for patients with AKI, and these values increase as AKI worsens.

AKI due to Contrast-Induced Nephropathy

Retrospective studies have reported a wide range of mortality rates for contrast-induced nephropathy (CIN): from a low of 1.1% to a high of 34% in patients who develop CIN after coronary angiography with or without percutaneous coronary intervention (PCI).[21] For patients with chronic renal insufficiency, the incidence of CIN rises to about 7%, and for patients with diabetes mellitus and chronic renal failure, it is greater than 50%.[22] Levy and colleagues demonstrated that patients who developed CIN had an adjusted odds ratio for death of 5.5.[23] Multiple interventions have been tested to reduce the risk of CIN, the most expensive of which is hemofiltration.[24] Klarenbach and coworkers performed a cost-effectiveness analysis and demonstrated that the ratio of cost to quality-adjusted life years (QALYs) gained favored the use of N-acetylcysteine, sodium bicarbonate, or saline.[25]

AKI Outcomes

Clearly, AKI in critically ill patients results from many different etiologies, as previously discussed. From a prognostic standpoint, the key to ensuring the best possible clinical and even health economic outcome is the expeditious and accurate recognition of the cause of the dysfunction. In the past, the term "acute renal failure" was used; however, it had multiple definitions and was linked with varying severities of illness. AKI represents a more rigorous and precise definition, and the severity of AKI is now stratified by either Risk–Injury–Failure–Loss–End Stage Renal Disease (RIFLE) or Acute Kidney Injury Network (AKIN) criteria, described in greater detail in other sources.[26,27] High AKI severity has been linked to poorer AKI-associated clinical outcomes and as one would surmise, the earlier detection of AKI may permit the institution of timely interventions that may improve patient outcomes and ultimately reduce costs.[26,28] Although no specific, definitive, and consensus treatment to reverse AKI exists, early detection nevertheless may ensure closer monitoring and even preemptive triage of patients to higher acuity settings such as ICUs or intermediate care/step-down units.

Three measurable outcomes regarding the effects of AKI include length of stay, progression to chronic kidney disease (CKD) or end-stage kidney disease, and mortality. From a health economic standpoint, Shaw and colleagues suggested that use of a novel biomarker for the diagnosis AKI may be cost effective when viewed from the societal perspective.[29] From the more basic standpoint regarding the level of resources consumed by patients with AKI, data from 23 Massachusetts hospitals over 2 years demonstrated that AKI resulted in higher hospital resource utilization, as both median direct hospital costs and hospital length of stay were increased by $2600 and by 5 days, respectively, in patients with AKI versus those without AKI.[30] Further, Chertow and colleagues demonstrated that even uncomplicated AKI was associated both with greater hospital costs and longer lengths of stay.[9] Although the length of stay may give some indication of the severity of patient illness and AKI, other factors such as concomitant organ dysfunction or hospital policies may affect this variable. Along with this, from a mortality standpoint, even after correcting for comorbidities, multiple studies have shown an increase in mortality associated with increasing RIFLE class.[31,32] However, mortality rates in AKI patients treated with RRT have improved over the past decade.[33,34]

The majority of patients surviving AKI recover renal function. However, a proportion of these patients subsequently develop CKD or end-stage kidney disease. The mechanisms for progression of AKI to CKD and end-stage kidney disease are unknown. Thirteen percent of patients in the BEST Kidney trial required RRT upon hospital discharge.[35] It is known that patients with preexisting CKD are more likely to develop end-stage kidney disease. Prescott and colleagues' database showed that 53% of patients with CKD developed end-stage kidney disease compared to only 13% of patients with normal baseline kidney function.[36] Chawla and coworkers suggested that advanced age, low serum albumin, diabetes, and severity of AKI (assessed by RIFLE score or mean serum creatinine) are predictive of poor renal outcomes.[37]

ACUTE TUBULAR NECROSIS

If AKI recognized too late in its course or if one is not able to reverse the process even in the case of expeditious diagnosis, then AKI may progress to acute tubular necrosis (ATN). In the ATN state, the glomerular filtration rate (GFR) is reduced to the point where drugs that are renally metabolized may have a prolonged presence and action. As a result, levels of drugs are often monitored, for which there is an added cost. During this period, fluid balance is carefully monitored with strict measurement of intake and output and controlled with diuretics, which may take the form of continuous drips in severe cases. The long-term sequelae of developing ATN is that up to 20% of patients progress to CKD stage 4 or greater within 18 to 24 months.[38]

Hemodialysis

When the effects of ATN (eg, acidemia, hyperkalemia, volume overload, uremia) cannot be controlled, patients are then often considered for RRT. According to Hoste and colleagues, 200 to 300 patients per million population who develop AKI each year require RRT.[39] Despite this intervention, these patients still have a mortality rate of 50% to 60%.[39]

RRT is either administered intermittently or continuously. Multiple studies (discussed later) indicate that intermittent hemodialysis (IHD) is less expensive with similar efficacy compared to continuous renal replacement therapy (CRRT).[40] If indications so warrant, hemodialysis can be performed daily and can be run for extended treatment times (6–8 hours), that is, slow low-efficiency daily dialysis (SLEDD). Similar cost savings are achieved with SLEDD.[41]

The determination of the best RRT approach that one should employ is dependent on a number of factors, including but not limited to staff and physician training, reimbursement systems, and the need for ongoing dialysis treatment. Trends have been changing from 1998 to 2005 regarding the use of CRRT, SLEDD, and IHD: CRRT was increasingly used for AKI, from 9.9% of patients in 1998 to 18.3% by 2005. The proportion of daily dialysis prescriptions also decreased during this period, while use of intermittent hemodialysis remained stable at approximately 68%.[42] Clearly then, high health care costs[40] and significant consumption of resources[43] are the norm in the care of patients with AKI.

Slow Low-Efficiency Daily Dialysis

Continuous therapies are usually preferred when either the patient is hemodynamically unstable and would not be able to maintain blood pressure given the high flows of hemodialysis or numerous interventions/situations require more precise fluid, acid–base, and electrolyte management. SLEDD is seen as a hybrid of IHD and CRRT. SLEDD is noted in the literature by various names: extended daily dialysis, sustained low-efficiency dialysis (SLED), and sustained low-efficiency daily diafiltration. Although the logistical mechanics regarding the use of SLEDD likely differ across the world, in the United States, SLEDD is typically delivered by hemodialysis nurses under the supervision of a nephrology specialist. This is in contrast to CRRT, which may be delivered by ICU nursing staff, although again variation is likely the norm. Solute clearance in CRRT (especially small and middle molecules) may benefit patients with AKI who are critically ill.[44,45] There have been speculations that large molecule removal may be beneficial in certain circumstances.[46,47] Even though intermittent therapies do not achieve the same clearances as continuous, when performed daily as in SLEDD, they are comparable. However, the differences in the clearance of various molecular substances may potentially make CRRT advantageous.

CRRT

Studies and papers have argued that CRRT is superior to intermittent hemodialysis.[48–50] Purported benefits include better control of fluid balance and hemodynamic stability. However, at least one study of patients with multiorgan dysfunction shows that either modality can be used effectively.[51] Vinsoneau showed in their multicenter trial that the rate of survival at 60 days did not differ between the intermittent hemodialysis group (32%) and the CRRT group (33%). A meta-analysis of nine randomized controlled trials (RCTs; published and unpublished) similarly showed that the initial choice of IHD versus CRRT did not affect mortality (odds ratio [OR], 0.99; 95% confidence interval [CI], 0.78–1.26).[52] Pannu and colleagues similarly found no difference in all-cause mortality in seven RCTs (relative risk [RR], 1.10; 95% CI, 0.99–1.23).[53]

Renal Recovery

If the ATN resolves in the ICU, then the patient's RRT is discontinued. However, many times ATN recovery time is prolonged beyond the need for ICU-level care. As a result, hemodialysis is continued outside of the ICU.

Although in-hospital survival of critically ill patients is poor and rarely exceeds 30%, the long-term survival of patients who leave the hospital is more promising. After discharge from the hospital, approximately 10% to 30% of patients who require the institution of RRT will require further dialysis treatment.[44,54,55] In a German study that investigated 979 patients in the ICU, the 6-month survival of patients who survived to hospital discharge was approximately 69% and the 5-year survival was 50%.[56] Of these patients, only 10% required chronic dialysis, and the renal function in the remaining 59% of the patients eventually returned to normal. Seventy-seven percent of surviving patients reported good-to-excellent health status. A prospective pilot study in patients in the ICU who had ARF and were treated with RRT found that mental and physical SF-36 health survey questionnaire scores at 6 months were similar to, or slightly lower than, those of the age-matched general population. Almost all patients stated that they would choose dialysis again.[57] Also, in this group, 73% of the patients who were discharged from the hospital survived 6 months. Bagshaw and colleagues performed a meta-analysis of four studies that noted that initial modality does not influence renal recovery independent of RRT (OR, 0.76; 95% CI, 0.28–2.07).[52] Pannu similarly found no difference in the requirement for chronic dialysis treatment in survivors (RR, 0.91; 95% CI, 0.56–1.49).[53] As the evidence for mortality and continued need for RRT grows, the debate regarding the superiority of one modality over another will continue.[58,59]

RESOURCES, COST STUDIES, AND ECONOMIC EVALUATIONS

The treatment of kidney disease in critically ill patients, as previously alluded to, consumes vast sums of scarce resources, and in view of limited budgets and heightened concerns regarding health care costs, it is vital to examine both the costs of care itself in conjunction with the associated outcomes and the inherent cost-effectiveness. The concept of limited resources, by definition, invokes the notion of opportunity costs, a perspective that at some level elevates the issue of cost and economics from the individual patient to the societal and public health realm. The patient's mortality, need for continued dialysis, and his or her quality of life are all important factors to consider when evaluating the effectiveness of a treatment. Aside from the direct costs associated with the specific treatment modalities for AKI and other renal diseases, the costs and resources utilized in the treatment of AKI may involve additional and often substantial indirect components including costs associated with nursing and custodial care care, increased length of ICU or hospital stay, and additional dialysis sessions. In addition, one also must consider the indirect but nevertheless substantial economic and quality of life issues associated with lost productivity, reduced quality of life, and related qualitative and quantitative aspects.

Accordingly, when measuring the costs associated with AKI treatment, one must consider both short-term and long-term direct costs. In addition, costs associated with adverse events (such as medication dosing, electrolyte management, fluid management, acid/base management, dietary management, etc) must also be considered. Depending on the outcome following AKI treatment, one may also need to incorporate the cost of continued outpatient hemodialysis if there is not renal recovery.

Financial Aspects of RRT for AKI

The literature contains multiple economic analyses of RRT for AKI. Few studies consider long-term consequences and costs related to RRT. Instead most focus on direct, short-term costs. Mehta, for example, compared the daily costs for continuous arterio/venovenous hemodiafiltration (CAVHDF/CVVHDF) to the costs for IHD.[60] Material costs were significantly higher for CRRT ($338) than for IHD ($66). The major components comprising the CRRT costs included the dialysate (33% of total cost), the filters (20%), and the rental costs of infusion pumps (20%). The labor costs for IHD were $216 and for CRRT $205. The total direct cost per treatment was $543 for CRRT and for IHD the total direct cost was $282. Although the daily cost for CRRT is more than that for IHD, the difference in costs is largely related to the increased expense of materials. At the time this study was done, CRRT was not as widely used as it is today, and the cost of materials has changed. In addition, the number of filter kits that are used can also influence the costs for CRRT. As CRRT techniques gain wider acceptance and methods to promote filter life are more universally adapted, it is likely that this difference in overall costs will be significantly reduced.

Vitale also compared daily costs of continuous and intermittent (4 hours daily) RRTs in an Italian single-center study.[61] In this study, the daily cost of CRRT was estimated at euro 276.70, of which 79% was for devices and 21% was for human resources. The daily cost of 4-hour IHD sessions was euro 247.83, of which 44% was for technical devices and 56% was for human resources. The expenditure for CRRT was 12% higher than that for IHDF owing to the cost of technical devices. However, in this study, IHD was used as a "bridge" between ICU CRRT and RRT in the dialysis unit. Given that the same machine is used to perform IHD/SLEDD as outpatient hemodialysis, it is understandable that the device cost is low. Depending on the arrangement, SLEDD and IHD are performed by a dedicated hemodialysis nurse for the duration of the treatment. Unless one's RRT arrangement is similar to that of Vitale, it is difficult to generalize their findings. However, there are reports of SLEDD being run by ICU nurses, reducing the additional need of a hemodialysis nurse.[62] Regarding their cost estimates, CRRT requires investment in a new machine for which ICU nurses are usually responsible to administer the continuous treatment. Usually cost estimates do not include nurse training time or the time necessary to troubleshoot the machine, for example, in cases of clotting. It is also difficult to assess the cost of nurse-related services, whether dialysis nurses (usually from a different department) or ICU nurse staff.

Rauf and coworkers examined the mean adjusted costs from the start of RRT to discharge.[63] In their study, after adjustment for differences in baseline patient characteristics (including severity of illness), the RRT method (IHD or CRRT) did not affect the likelihood of renal recovery, in-hospital survival, or survival during follow-up. In this two tertiary care center trail of 161 patients, mean adjusted ICU length of stay was 9.5 days shorter for IHD-treated than CRRT-treated patients ($P<.001$), and the adjusted mean differences in hospital and total costs associated with ICU stay were $56,564 and $60,827, respectively, in favor of IHD ($P<.001$). Examining total costs more closely, IHD costs were on average $51,556 less for treatment of ARF compared with CRRT-treated patients (CRRT, $106,377 vs IHD, $54,821; 95% CI of difference, $20,749–$82,363). The authors also demonstrated significantly reduced hospital ($47,405; $P = .001$) and physician ($4152; $P = .001$) costs for IHD-treated patients during ICU stay. They attribute this to reduced dialysis, pharmacy, and laboratory-related costs among IHD versus CRRT patients (pharmacy costs CRRT, $18,486 vs IHD, $6,768; $P<.001$). Mean adjusted total costs through hospital discharge were $93,611 and $140,733 among IHD-treated and CRRT-treated patients, respectively ($P<.001$). A closer look at this study shows that patients receiving CRRT received significantly higher amounts of mechanical ventilation, and inotropic support, were oliguric, and were more likely to have a DNR/DNI code status. Although patients with higher APACHE II scores contributed to higher costs of care, when adjusting for the severity of illness, CRRT still was determined to be more costly.[63]

CRRT requires frequent electrolyte monitoring and replacement when necessary. Disposable costs in CRRT are higher: filter costs are higher and are more likely to be replaced compared to during IHD treatments. With the low blood flow rates in CRRT, anticoagulation may also be necessary. However, some machines are able to achieve faster blood flows, making anticoagulation less of an issue.

Srisawat and colleagues estimated RRT costs from the BEST Kidney study, a multicenter observational study from 2000–2001 including data from 23 countries.[64] Theorized hospital costs for staffing, dialysate and replacement fluid, anticoagulation, and the extracorporeal circuit ranged from $3,629.80/day more with CRRT to $378.60/day more with intermittent RRT. The costs were highly variable from center to center, with some institutions demonstrating lower costs with CRRT. This analysis suggests that there may be institutional factors that must be accounted for when assessing the costs of each modality. For example, this study concluded that CRRT costs may be reduced by limiting the CRRT solution rates to 25 mL/min or less. The authors argued this would reduce fluid costs by 43% and total CRRT costs by 19.5%. Delivery standards have changed since 2000, and this study used theoretical costs developed from a retrospective study. Also, this study compared countries of differing economic development status, which may lead to the wide ranges in costs.

SLEDD Versus CRRT

In an observational, prospective pilot study, Berbece and coworkers attempted to describe the costs specially attributed to SLED compared to CRRT (CVVHD/CVVHDF).[41] In this study, SLED consisted of 8 hours of HD 6 days a week, with blood flow of 200 mL/min, dialysate flows of 350 mL/min, and hemofiltration of 60 mL/min. Equivalent clearance was achieved with each modality. This single center Canadian experience demonstrated lower costs with SLEDD compared to CRRT: $1431 for SLED, $2607 for CRRT with heparin, and $3089 for CRRT with citrate. Incremental single treatment, per patient cost in this study was $170. One week of SLEDD treatment performed by an hempdialysis nurse would increase costs by $2450. In this study, this was similar to the cost of CRRT with heparin, but still less than that of CRRT with citrate anticoagulation.

Klarenbach and coworkers developed a Markov model to compare the costs of daily IHD, SLEDD, and standard and high-dose CRRT.[65] This cost-utility analysis started with the base-case assumption that CRRT was associated with similar health outcomes but higher costs by ($3679 more than IHD per patient). The authors noted that a sensitivity analysis demonstrated that mortality and need for long-term RRT would alter the cost-effectiveness for any modality. The authors concluded that IHD was the most attractive modality given a choice between IHD and CRRT.

Development of a CRRT Program

As of this writing, the approximate cost for the machine is $30,000 each, cartridges are $160/each, solutions average $25.00 per 5-L bag (personal communications, 2011). In the study of Berbece and coworkers, the filter/tubing set for CRRT cost $185, whereas the filter and tubing for SLED cost $35.60.[41] Solutions in their study for CRRT cost either $5.50/L (Hemosol BO) or $7.70/L (Normocarb), whereas dialysate produced for SLED cost about $0.09/L.[41] Maintenance for the machine averages $3000 per machine per year. Nursing costs are highly variable based on the region and the arrangement of delivery. Specific to the treatment time, dialysis nurses can average $20 to $40 per hour, whereas the rates for ICU nurses are higher. ICU nurses are also responsible for other aspects of patient care during the delivery of CRRT, whereas the dialysis nurse is focused only on the delivery of the treatment. As a result of the increased amount of patient attention required for patients receiving CRRT, ICU nurses are often placed in a 1:1 patient-to-nurse ratio. The model of delivery is important at the initiation of a CRRT program and may have future cost implications.[66,67] In the study of Berbece and colleagues, the average daily cost of CRRT with regional citrate anticoagulation was $440, and for CRRT with heparin it was $335.[41] Citrate is currently not FDA approved for regional anticoagulation and is currently more expensive than heparin.

Gilbert and colleagues determined the costs associated with starting a CRRT program in critically ill patients at $79,622.[68] However, it is difficult to assess the appropriate context of this, because ultimately the issue is not one of cost but rather cost-effectiveness, in terms of the joint assessment of clinical outcome relative to costs and resources that are expended. To date, no randomized clinical trial has demonstrated a benefit of early dialysis initiation versus late initiation. No RCT has shown benefit of one modality over another. Limitations of these studies include design issues such as sample size and randomization. A few studies have addressed the question of dose of dialysis but a number of them are not comparable to one another. One major difference between the studies is the type of therapy: convective, diffusive, or both. Renal function recovery has been suggested with CRRT, and hemodynamic stability is also another advantage. In addition, there are a number of nonrenal-related applications and support that CRRT offers. The ideal modality in the ICU preserves homeostasis without sacrificing the treatment of comorbidities or the patient's underlying condition.[69] In addition the modality should be simple to manage and not burdensome to the staff. The complexity of CRRT therapy, lack of well trained nurses and physicians, significant start-up and maintenance costs, and a history of low reimbursement are all significant barriers to implementation. Despite these added costs, Hoyt argued that the advantages of better nutrition, fluid balance, hemodynamic management, and renal recovery make up for the difference.[70]

In the aforementioned studies it is difficult to determine whether one modality is more expensive than the other. Some authors may include costs that others do not. Nursing ratios (1:1 vs 1:2) and whether there is a role for the dialysis nurse changes the cost perspective. Anticoagulation will affect the survival of the filter, the rate of and need for replacement solutions, and the frequency of laboratory tests.

Cost reduction potential is apparent in numerous areas including dialysis access and anticoagulation regimens, dose of dialysis (ie, the amount of dialysate and replacement solutions used), and ensuring the appropriate patient is selected for treatment.

Role of Biomarkers to Predict the Need for RRT and Chances of Recovery

The potential role of biomarkers in this area is growing. Biomarkers such as neutrophil gelatinase–associated lipocalin (NGAL) and cystatin C can be used to identify patients earlier, which potentially may reduce the severity of AKI.[4,71] Parikh and colleagues showed that a cost savings can be realized by utilizing NGAL to identify AKI in the emergency room setting.[72] The other potential application of biomarkers would be to use them to determine the severity of AKI and whether RRT will become necessary. This will add an interesting twist to the early-versus-late initiation of RRT debate. Lastly, biomarkers may be able to predict whether a patient will realize renal recovery or not. This would improve disposition planning and may reduce the inpatient resources currently utilized while awaiting a sign of recovery. These biomarker applications are largely speculative at this time.

SUMMARY

Although multiple studies explore the consequences and costs of AKI and its treatments, the main cost of AKI is due to the long-term progression to CKD. Progression to CKD requires the follow-up of a nephrologist and health care expenditures to prevent progression to end-stage renal disease. At present, approximately one third of patients with AKI requiring dialysis see a nephrologist within 30 days of discharge.[37] This CKD population, especially persons with stages 4 to 5, has low quality of life and estimates of utility.[73,74] This long-term cost, and ultimately the cost-effectiveness of AKI, still must be explored.

REFERENCES

1. Hou SH, Bushinsky DA, Wish JB, et al. Hospital-acquired renal insufficiency: a prospective study. Am J Med 1983;74(2):243–8.
2. Nash K, Hafeez A, Hou S. Hospital-acquired renal insufficiency. Am J Kidney Dis 2002;39(5):930–6.
3. Shusterman N, Strom BL, Murray TG, et al. Risk factors and outcome of hospital-acquired acute renal failure: clinical epidemiologic study. Am J Med 1987;83(1): 65–71.
4. Nickolas TL, Barasch J, Devarajan P. Biomarkers in acute and chronic kidney disease. Curr Opin Nephrol Hypertens 2008;17(2):127–32.
5. Uchino S, Kellum JA, Bellomo R, et al. Acute renal failure in critically ill patients: a multinational, multicenter study. JAMA 2005;294(7):813–8.
6. Chertow GM, Soroko SH, Paganini EP, et al. Mortality after acute renal failure: models for prognostic stratification and risk adjustment. Kidney Int 2006;70(6):1120–6.
7. Bellomo R. The epidemiology of acute renal failure: 1975 versus 2005. Curr Opin Crit Care 2006;12(6):557–60.
8. Ympa YP, Sakr Y, Reinhart K, et al. Has mortality from acute renal failure decreased? A systematic review of the literature. Am J Med 2005;118(8):827–32.
9. Chertow GM, Burdick E, Honour M, et al. Acute kidney injury, mortality, length of stay, and costs in hospitalized patients. J Am Soc Nephrol 2005;16(11):3365–70.

10. Langenberg C, Wan L, Egi M, et al. Renal blood flow in experimental septic acute renal failure. Kidney Int 2006;69(11):1996–2002.

11. Brenner M, Schaer GL, Mallory DL, et al. Detection of renal blood flow abnormalities in septic and critically ill patients using a newly designed indwelling thermodilution renal vein catheter. Chest 1990;98(1):170–9.

12. Bagshaw SM, Uchino S, Bellomo R, et al. Septic acute kidney injury in critically ill patients: clinical characteristics and outcomes. Clin J Am Soc Nephrol 2007;2(3): 431–9.

13. Neveu H, Kleinknecht D, Brivet F, et al. and The French Study Group on Acute Renal Failure. Prognostic factors in acute renal failure due to sepsis. Results of a prospective multicentre study. Nephrol Dial Transplant 1996;11(2):293–9.

14. Lassnigg A, Schmidlin D, Mouhieddine M, et al. Minimal changes of serum creatinine predict prognosis in patients after cardiothoracic surgery: a prospective cohort study. J Am Soc Nephrol 2004;15(6):1597–605.

15. Dasta JF, Kane-Gill SL, Durtschi AJ, et al. Costs and outcomes of acute kidney injury (AKI) following cardiac surgery. Nephrol Dial Transplant 2008;23(6):1970–4.

16. Kuitunen A, Vento A, Suojaranta-Ylinen R, et al. Acute renal failure after cardiac surgery: evaluation of the RIFLE classification. Ann Thorac Surg 2006;81(2):542–6.

17. Hoste EA, Cruz DN, Davenport A, et al. The epidemiology of cardiac surgery-associated acute kidney injury. Int J Artif Organs 2008;31(2):158–65.

18. Leacche M, Rawn JD, Mihaljevic T, et al. Outcomes in patients with normal serum creatinine and with artificial renal support for acute renal failure developing after coronary artery bypass grafting. Am J Cardiol 2004;93(3):353–6.

19. Mehta RH, Grab JD, O'Brien SM, et al. Bedside tool for predicting the risk of postoperative dialysis in patients undergoing cardiac surgery. Circulation 21 2006; 114(21):2208–16 [quiz: 2208].

20. Callahan M, Battleman DS, Christos P, et al. Economic consequences of renal dysfunction among cardiopulmonary bypass surgery patients: a hospital-based perspective. Value Health 2003;6(2):137–43.

21. Rudnick M, Feldman H. Contrast-induced nephropathy: what are the true clinical consequences? Clin J Am Soc Nephrol 2008;3(1):263–72.

22. McCullough PA, Wolyn R, Rocher LL, et al. Acute renal failure after coronary intervention: incidence, risk factors, and relationship to mortality. Am J Med 1997; 103(5):368–75.

23. Levy EM, Viscoli CM, Horwitz RI. The effect of acute renal failure on mortality: a cohort analysis. JAMA 1996;275(19):1489–94.

24. Marenzi G, Marana I, Lauri G, et al. The prevention of radiocontrast-agent-induced nephropathy by hemofiltration. N Engl J Med 2003;349(14):1333–40.

25. Klarenbach SW, Pannu N, Tonelli MA, et al. Cost-effectiveness of hemofiltration to prevent contrast nephropathy in patients with chronic kidney disease. Crit Care Med 2006;34(4):1044–51.

26. Bellomo R, Ronco C, Kellum JA, et al. Acute renal failure—definition, outcome measures, animal models, fluid therapy and information technology needs: the Second International Consensus Conference of the Acute Dialysis Quality Initiative (ADQI) Group. Crit Care 2004;8(4):R204–12.

27. Mehta RL, Kellum JA, Shah SV, et al. Acute Kidney Injury Network: report of an initiative to improve outcomes in acute kidney injury. Crit Care 2007;11(2):R31.

28. Uchino S, Bellomo R, Goldsmith D, et al. An assessment of the RIFLE criteria for acute renal failure in hospitalized patients. Crit Care Med 2006;34(7):1913–7.

29. Shaw A, Chalfin D. Economic impact and cost-effectiveness of urine neutrophil gelatinase-associated lipocalin following cardiac surgery. Crit Care 2010; 14(Suppl 1):530.

30. Fischer MJ, Brimhall BB, Lezotte DC, et al. Uncomplicated acute renal failure and hospital resource utilization: a retrospective multicenter analysis. Am J Kidney Dis 2005;46(6):1049–57.

31. Hoste EA, Clermont G, Kersten A, et al. RIFLE criteria for acute kidney injury are associated with hospital mortality in critically ill patients: a cohort analysis. Crit Care 2006;10(3):R73.

32. Uchino S, Bellomo R, Goldsmith D, et al. An assessment of the RIFLE criteria for acute renal failure in hospitalized patients. Crit Care Med 2006;34(7):1913–7.

33. Waikar SS, Curhan GC, Wald R, et al. Declining mortality in patients with acute renal failure, 1988 to 2002. J Am Soc Nephrol 2006;17(4):1143–50.

34. Xue JL, Daniels F, Star RA, et al. Incidence and mortality of acute renal failure in Medicare beneficiaries, 1992 to 2001. J Am Soc Nephrol 2006;17(4):1135–42.

35. Uchino S, Kellum JA, Bellomo R, et al. Acute renal failure in critically ill patients: a multinational, multicenter study. JAMA 2005;294(7):813–8.

36. Prescott GJ, Metcalfe W, Baharani J, et al. A prospective national study of acute renal failure treated with RRT: incidence, aetiology and outcomes. Nephrol Dial Transplant 2007;22(9):2513–9.

37. Chawla LS, Amdur RL, Amodeo S, et al. The severity of acute kidney injury predicts progression to chronic kidney disease. Kidney Int 2011;79(12):1361–9.

38. Amdur RL, Chawla LS, Amodeo S, et al. Outcomes following diagnosis of acute renal failure in U.S. veterans: focus on acute tubular necrosis. Kidney Int 2009;76(10): 1089–97.

39. Hoste EA, Schurgers M. Epidemiology of acute kidney injury: how big is the problem? Crit Care Med 2008;36(4 Suppl):S146–51.

40. Manns B, Doig CJ, Lee H, et al. Cost of acute renal failure requiring dialysis in the intensive care unit: clinical and resource implications of renal recovery. Crit Care Med 2003;31(2):449–55.

41. Berbece AN, Richardson RM. Sustained low-efficiency dialysis in the ICU: cost, anticoagulation, and solute removal. Kidney Int 2006;70(5):963–8.

42. Afshinnia F, Straight A, Li Q, et al. Trends in dialysis modality for individuals with acute kidney injury. Ren Fail 2009;31(8):647–54.

43. Hamel MB, Phillips RS, Davis RB, et al. and SUPPORT Investigators (Study to Understand Prognoses and Preferences for Outcomes and Risks of Treatments). Outcomes and cost-effectiveness of initiating dialysis and continuing aggressive care in seriously ill hospitalized adults. Ann Intern Med 1997;127(3):195–202.

44. Ronco C, Bellomo R, Homel P, et al. Effects of different doses in continuous veno-venous haemofiltration on outcomes of acute renal failure: a prospective randomised trial. Lancet 2000;356(9223):26–30.

45. Schiffl H, Lang SM, Fischer R. Daily hemodialysis and the outcome of acute renal failure. N Engl J Med 2002;346(5):305–10.

46. Schetz M. Non-renal indications for continuous renal replacement therapy. Kidney Int 1999;72(Suppl):S88–94.

47. Ronco C, Brendolan A, Bellomo R. Continuous versus intermittent renal replacement therapy in the treatment of acute renal failure. Nephrol Dial Transplant. 1998;13(Suppl 6):79–85.

48. Uchino S, Bellomo R, Ronco C. Intermittent versus continuous renal replacement therapy in the ICU: impact on electrolyte and acid-base balance. Intensive Care Med 2001;27(6):1037–43.

49. Ronco C, Bellomo R. Dialysis in intensive care unit patients with acute kidney injury: continuous therapy is superior. Clin J Am Soc Nephrol 2007;2(3):597–600.
50. Ronco C. Continuous dialysis is superior to intermittent dialysis in acute kidney injury of the critically ill patient. Nat Clin Pract Nephrol 2007;3(3):118–9.
51. Vinsonneau C, Camus C, Combes A, et al. Continuous venovenous haemodiafiltration versus intermittent haemodialysis for acute renal failure in patients with multiple-organ dysfunction syndrome: a multicentre randomised trial. Lancet 2006;368(9533): 379–85.
52. Bagshaw SM, Berthiaume LR, Delaney A, et al. Continuous versus intermittent renal replacement therapy for critically ill patients with acute kidney injury: a meta-analysis. Crit Care Med 2008;36(2):610–7.
53. Pannu N, Klarenbach S, Wiebe N, et al. Renal replacement therapy in patients with acute renal failure: a systematic review. JAMA 2008;299(7):793–805.
54. Cole L, Bellomo R, Silvester W, et al. A prospective, multicenter study of the epidemiology, management, and outcome of severe acute renal failure in a "closed" ICU system. Am J Respir Crit Care Med 2000;162(1):191–6.
55. Silvester W, Bellomo R, Cole L. Epidemiology, management, and outcome of severe acute renal failure of critical illness in Australia. Crit Care Med 2001;29(10):1910–5.
56. Morgera S, Kraft AK, Siebert G, et al. Long-term outcomes in acute renal failure patients treated with continuous renal replacement therapies. Am J Kidney Dis 2002;40(2):275–9.
57. Maynard SE, Whittle J, Chelluri L, et al. Quality of life and dialysis decisions in critically ill patients with acute renal failure. Intensive Care Med 2003;29(9):1589–93.
58. Ronco C, Bagshaw SM, Gibney RT, et al. Outcome comparisons of intermittent and continuous therapies in acute kidney injury: what do they mean? Int J Artif Organs 2008;31(3):213–20.
59. Himmelfarb J. Continuous dialysis is not superior to intermittent dialysis in acute kidney injury of the critically ill patient. Nat Clin Pract Nephrol 2007;3(3):120–1.
60. Mehta RL, McDonald B, Gabbai FB, et al. A randomized clinical trial of continuous versus intermittent dialysis for acute renal failure. Kidney Int 2001;60(3):1154–63.
61. Vitale C, Bagnis C, Marangella M, et al. Cost analysis of blood purification in intensive care units: continuous versus intermittent hemodiafiltration. J Nephrol 2003;16(4): 572–9.
62. Marshall MR, Ma T, Galler D, et al. Sustained low-efficiency daily diafiltration (SLEDD-f) for critically ill patients requiring renal replacement therapy: towards an adequate therapy. Nephrol Dial Transplant 2004;19(4):877–84.
63. Rauf AA, Long KH, Gajic O, et al. Intermittent hemodialysis versus continuous renal replacement therapy for acute renal failure in the intensive care unit: an observational outcomes analysis. J Intensive Care Med 2008;23(3):195–203.
64. Srisawat N, Lawsin L, Uchino S, et al. Cost of acute renal replacement therapy in the intensive care unit: results from The Beginning and Ending Supportive Therapy for the Kidney (BEST Kidney) study. Crit Care 2010;14(2):R46.
65. Klarenbach S, Manns B, Pannu N, et al. Economic evaluation of continuous renal replacement therapy in acute renal failure. Int J Technol Assess Health Care 2009; 25(3):331–8.
66. Giuliano KK, Pysznik EE. Renal replacement therapy in critical care: implementation of a unit-based continuous venovenous hemodialysis program. Crit Care Nurs 1998; 18(1):40–51.
67. Ellis K. Who should provide continuous renal replacement therapies? Nephrology nurses are better prepared to provide CRRT. Nephrol Nurs J 2007;34(2):228–9.

68. Gilbert RW, Caruso DM, Foster KN, et al. Development of a continuous renal replacement program in critically ill patients. Am J Surg 2002;184(6):526–32 [discussion: 532–3].
69. Lameire N, Van Biesen W, Vanholder R. Dialysing the patient with acute renal failure in the ICU: the emperor's clothes? Nephrol Dial Transplant 1999;14(11):2570–3.
70. Hoyt DB. CRRT in the area of cost containment: is it justified? Am J Kidney Dis 1997;30(5 Suppl 4):S102–4.
71. Haase M, Bellomo R, Devarajan P, et al. Accuracy of neutrophil gelatinase-associated lipocalin (NGAL) in diagnosis and prognosis in acute kidney injury: a systematic review and meta-analysis. Am J Kidney Dis 2009;54(6):1012–24.
72. Parikh A, Rizzo J, Chalfin D, et al. Does NGAL reduce costs? A cost analysis of urine NGAL (uNGAL) & serum creatinine (SCr) for acute kidney injury (AKI) diagnosis. Crit Care Med 2010;38(12 Suppl):[abstract 390].
73. Gorodetskaya I, Zenios S, McCulloch CE, et al. Health-related quality of life and estimates of utility in chronic kidney disease. Kidney Int 2005;68(6):2801–8.
74. Perlman RL, Finkelstein FO, Liu L, et al. Quality of life in chronic kidney disease (CKD): a cross-sectional analysis in the Renal Research Institute-CKD study. Am J Kidney Dis 2005;45(4):658–66.

Economic and Outcomes Aspects of Venous Thromboembolic Disease

Chee M. Chan, MD, MPH*, Andrew F. Shorr, MD, MPH

KEYWORDS
- Venous thromboembolism • Cost • Economics
- Pulmonary embolism • Prevention
- Deep venous thrombosis

Venous thromboembolic (VTE) disease is associated with significant morbidity and mortality, particularly in critically ill patients. Preexisting impairments in both cardiac and pulmonary function limit the ability of these organs to compensate for an acute pulmonary embolus (PE). Risk factors associated with VTE vary depending on the reason for critical illness. For example, approximately 60% of patients admitted with a traumatic insult will develop a deep venous thrombosis (DVT)[1] compared to 28% to 32% in the general medical-surgical intensive care unit (ICU) population.[2,3] More concerning, the incidence of DVT is as high as 70% in acute stroke patients where 1% to 2% of patients with hemiplegia eventually succumb to a fatal PE.[4–6] The clinical status of ICU patients adds to the challenge of diagnosing VTE. Altered mental status, the use of sedatives, and intubation often mask clinical symptoms that may suggest VTE. Illustrating this, 95% of DVTs in the ICU are clinically silent.[7] Further, limitations in physiologic reserve of critically ill patients reduce their tolerability of not just the VTE, but also render these subjects poor candidates for full-dose anticoagulation. Patients in the ICU are often at increased risk for bleeding and are unlikely to tolerate bleeding should it occur.[8] Thus, in combination these factors emphasize the need to effectively prevent VTE in this setting.

The potentially devastating consequences associated with VTE in the ICU can also have profound financial implications. This healthcare burden is not just limited to the acute inpatient stay but also extends into the need for closer outpatient care. As a consequence, from a healthcare as well as a financial standpoint, the importance of preventing VTE has led the American College of Chest Physicians (ACCP) to make prevention guidelines to enhance efforts to reduce VTE risk. These guidelines underscore

The authors have nothing to disclose.

Division of Pulmonary and Critical Care Medicine, Department of Medicine, Washington Hospital Center, 110 Irving Street NW, No. 2B-39, Washington, DC 20010, USA

* Corresponding author.

E-mail address: chee262@hotmail.com

Crit Care Clin 28 (2012) 113–123

doi:10.1016/j.ccc.2011.09.005

criticalcare.theclinics.com

the need for clinicians to carefully weigh the risk:benefit ratio of thromboprophylaxis in this high-risk group. However, to fully understand the financial scope of this disease in the ICU, one must first understand (1) the epidemiology of VTE in the ICU, (2) the risk factors associated with the development of VTE, (3) treatment options, and (4) the healthcare policy regarding VTE prophylaxis.

EPIDEMIOLOGY OF VTE IN THE ICU

DVT is the predominant presentation of VTE in the ICU. However, as a small component of a larger spectrum of disease, namely VTE, one must understand the close relationship between DVT and PE. In the general medical population, approximately 40% to 50% of patients with symptomatic proximal DVT will also have a concurrent asymptomatic PE on screening examination.[9,10] Conversely, of the general medical patients admitted with a PE, 70% to 80% will have a concomitant DVT.[11]

In general, the epidemiology of PE in the ICU is not well understood. Establishing the incidence of PE in an ICU presents challenges since the diagnostic modalities available for PE are limited in these subjects. The risk for contrast nephropathy from chest computed tomography (CT) in a population likely to have concurrent impaired renal function due to critical illness precludes screening for PE in the ICU. Further, the inability of intubated patients to cognitively make an inspiratory effort limits the use of ventilation/perfusion scintigraphy (V/Q scan). Thus, most epidemiologic data regarding PE in the ICU derive from autopsy data. Among autopsies performed in critically ill patients, about 7% to 27% have an incidental PE with an estimated 1% to 3% being fatal.[12–17] However, one must interpret postmortem data carefully because there is substantial selection bias—autopsies tend to be performed predominantly when cause of death is uncertain. Lack of uniformity in performing postmortem examinations restricts our understanding of the true mortality rate attributable to PE. In fact, only about 6% to 8% of ICU patients will ever have an autopsy performed.[18] Further, there is a 20% to 45% discrepancy rate between premortem and postmortem diagnoses in the ICU, which raises concern about diagnostic accuracy in critically ill patients.[16,19,20] Unfortunately, PE represents one of the top 3 major diagnoses that are most frequently missed in the ICU.[16,18,19]

Similarly, few clinical studies have evaluated the incidence of VTE in the critically ill. One of the first studies was performed by Moser and colleagues and involved 34 patients admitted to a respiratory ICU.[12] They conducted a prospective observational trial where 23 of the 34 participants underwent radiofibrinogen leg scans within the first week of admission. Of these, 13% were found to be abnormal indicating the presence of DVT. In a more recent larger prospective observation study, 261 patients admitted to a medical-surgical ICU had screening bilateral lower extremity compression ultrasonography performed within 48 hours of admission, then twice weekly until discharge from the ICU.[21] Within the first 48 hours, 2.7% of patients were diagnosed with a DVT. These findings demonstrate that ICU patients are extremely hypercoagulable even on admission to the ICU. Additionally, the use of serial lower extremity Duplex ultrasonography revealed that approximately 30% of the general medical-surgical ICU patient population will develop a DVT.[2] Multiple studies further document that DVT tends to occur within the first week of hospitalization in the ICU. In one particular study, 24% of DVT arose within the first week and further illustrates the importance of expeditious assessment for and administration of thromboprophylaxis in this patient population.[21]

Ibrahim and colleagues also evaluated the incidence of PE in those diagnosed with DVT in a prospective cohort study.[22] In 110 ventilated medical ICU patients, 23.6% developed DVT despite 100% employment of thromboprophylaxis. To qualify for enrollment, all subjects were mechanically ventilated for a minimum of 7 days and had screening lower extremity Doppler ultrasounds performed for the diagnosis of DVT. When a DVT was diagnosed, the incidence of PE was 11.5% compared to 0% when DVT was not diagnosed ($P = .012$).

RISK FACTORS ASSOCIATED WITH VTE IN THE ICU

Given the difficulties in diagnosing VTE in the ICU, awareness of the risk factors associated with VTE may increase one's clinical suspicion and, in turn, the likelihood for diagnosis. Three fundamental principles predispose individuals to clot formation: injury to the vascular endothelium, an alternation in the constitution of the blood or a hypercoagulable state, and a disturbance to normal blood flow or stasis.[9] Known as Virchow's triad, these principles explain the majority of risk factors associated with higher rates of VTE.

The ICU patient population possesses a unique set of characteristics that predispose them to thrombosis. Not only do they possess the same VTE risk factors as the general medical population, but they also have ICU acquired risk factors as well. Risk factors that contribute to the increased risk for hospital acquired VTE in the general medical population include age greater than 75 years, immobilization, the performance of procedures, and the presence of certain comorbid conditions, such as congestive heart failure, acute infection, and malignancy. Moreover, multiple randomized controlled therapeutic trials have verified that hospitalized patients often have more than one risk factor for hypercoagulability, and that these factors have an additive effect. In the Prophylaxis in Medical Patients with Enoxaparin (MEDENOX) study,[23] where over 1100 subjects were enrolled, factors that were independently associated with higher rates of in-hospital VTE included age greater than 75 years, the presence of an active infection, the presence of a malignancy, and a prior history of VTE. On average, those enrolled in MEDENOX had more than 2 risk factors. These findings were subsequently confirmed in 2 other large randomized trials: the Prospective Evaluation of Dalteparin Efficacy for Prevention of VTE in Immobilized Patients Trial (PREVENT)[24] and the Arixtra for Thromboembolism Prevention in a Medical Indications Study (ARTEMIS).[25]

In addition to these risk factors, prolonged immobilization due to mechanical ventilation, sedation, and/or hemodynamic instability represent a central ICU-acquired risk factor. These issues uniformly affect all ICU subjects, regardless of the admitting diagnosis.[26] Simultaneously, the need for invasive tests and procedures, such as central line placement, increase the likelihood for developing a VTE.[22] Most important, specific diagnoses that tend to occur often in the ICU also heighten the risk for VTE. For example, sepsis activates the coagulation cascade while trauma causes injury to the vascular endothelium, rendering these 2 populations very susceptible to thrombus formation. Other risk factors that are associated with thrombogenesis include the diagnosis of stroke, the diagnosis of an acute myocardial infarction,[9] and the use of vasopressors.[21]

THROMBOPROPHYLAXIS RECOMMENDATIONS

Unlike the surgical literature, the evidence for thromboprophylaxis in the critically ill patient is quite limited. Variability in the patient population warrants individualized risk assessment for VTE while simultaneously considering the bleeding risks. In general, there are 2 forms of VTE prophylaxis: chemical and mechanical. Pharmacological VTE prophylaxis is usually the preferred modality for thromboprophylaxis in the ICU. Although still limited, the data supporting chemical anticoagulants are more robust in this particular cohort. There are several effective pharmacologic agents available for critical care patients such as unfractionated heparin (UFH) and low-molecular-weight heparins (LMWH) like dalteparin and enoxaparin. Anti-Xa compounds, such as fondaparinux, have demonstrated safety and efficacy in the general medical population, but there are currently no data supporting their use in the ICU. Thus far, only 3 randomized controlled trials (RCTs) have been performed to evaluate the safety and efficacy of thromboprophylaxis in critical care patients. In the first study, Cade and colleagues randomized 119 critically ill patients to UFH 5000 U twice daily versus placebo.[2] All patients had daily ^{125}I-labeled fibrinogen leg scans to evaluate the incidence of DVT. The incidence of DVT was 13% in the group who received UFH compared to 29% in the placebo group with a relative risk reduction of 55% ($P<.05$). The investigators also randomized another 131 general medical patients and noted that only about 10% of these patients developed DVT when thromboprophylaxis was not prescribed. Thus, based on the findings of this study, ICU patients have at least 3 times the risk of developing VTE compared to the general medical patient.

In the second RCT, 223 mechanically ventilated patients with chronic obstructive pulmonary disease (COPD) were randomized to an LMWH, nadoparin, versus placebo.[3] LMWH is a short-chain polysaccharide produced by fractionation or depolymerization of UFH. Doppler ultrasonography was performed upon enrollment into the study, weekly, and when clinical DVT was suspected. Further, every patient had venography performed upon completion of the study, after early discontinuation from the study, or as a confirmatory test after a positive or indeterminant Doppler ultrasound result. The primary outcome was the incidence of DVT, and the secondary outcome measure was the rate of adverse effects (eg, major bleeding, minor bleeding, and thrombocytopenia associated with DVT prophylaxis). The use of nadoparin significantly reduced the incidence of DVT from 28.2% to 15.5% ($P = .045$). There was also no difference in the rate of adverse events (46.3% for nadoparin compared to 39.8% for placebo; $P = .33$). Thus, LMWH is both safe and efficacious for the prevention of DVT in mechanically ventilated ICU patients.

The third RCT, the Prophylaxis for Thrombeombolism in Critical Care Trial (PROTECT), assigned 3764 critically ill medical-surgical patients to either UFH or a LMWH, dalteparin to evaluate the superiority of dalteparin 5000 U once daily over UFH 5000 U twice daily while in the ICU.[27] Unique because of its size and use of an active comparator, in this trial Doppler ultrasonography was performed within 48 hours of admission and twice weekly to assess the proximal venous system for DVT. When clinically indicated, further imaging was performed to evaluate for symptomatic acute PE. The primary outcome was the incidence of DVT (both clinically evident and silent) while the secondary outcomes included any DVT, PE, VTE, or death. Additional secondary outcomes comprised the rate of major bleeding and heparin induced thrombocytopenia (HIT). The incidence rate of DVT was similar between both groups: 5.1% for dalteparin and 5.8% for UFH, $P = .57$. Interestingly, there were more PEs observed with UFH (2.3%) compared to dalteparin (1.3%, $P = .01$). From a safety standpoint, the risk of bleeding and the development of HIT did not differ between the two agents. Major bleeding occurred in 5.5% of those who received dalteparin versus 5.6% of those who received UFH ($P = .98$), while HIT was confirmed in only 0.3% of subjects assigned to dalteparin and in 0.6% who were assigned to UFH ($P = .16$). Thus, the utilization of DVT prophylaxis in the ICU can successfully and safely decrease the rate of VTE to approximately 5%. The ability of these agents to successfully prevent VTE with minimal rates of adverse events is necessary to protect ICU patients from the sequelae of developing a VTE: worsening hemodynamics, worsening respiratory status, and even death. Given the potentially devastating consequences of withholding VTE prophylaxis in this patient population, standardization of thromboprophylaxis is paramount in the ICU.

Several prospective observational trials have elucidated how the development of VTE in the ICU affects patient outcomes. One such trial enrolled 261 medical surgical critical care patients where 98% of patients received some form of DVT prophylaxis: 92.8% received UFH 5000 U twice daily and 7.2% received mechanical prophylaxis.[21] Akin to the PROTECT trial, screening for DVT was done within 48 hours of admission to the ICU, then twice weekly thereafter or when the physician was concerned about DVT based on signs and symptoms. DVT was assessed using bilateral lower extremity Doppler ultrasonography and the diagnosis of PE was sought when clinically indicated. Despite the high rate of thromboprophylaxis, the incidence of DVT was 9.6% (95% confidence interval [CI], 6.3 to 13.8) and of these cases, 9.4% developed a symptomatic PE. Mechanical ventilation days were significantly increased when VTE occurred (9 vs 6 days, $P = .03$), indicating both clear and substantial morbidity and resource use penalty related to ICU-acquired PE There were, however, several limitations in this report. As a prospective observational cohort study, it lacked a control group to facilitate clear comparisons. In fact, the higher incidence of DVT despite DVT prophylaxis raises the question of whether this finding is due to prophylaxis failure versus patient selection, particularly given the mixed medical-surgical population enrolled. Further, the diagnostic accuracy of Doppler ultrasonography has never been confirmed in ICU patients, and thus, the incidence of DVT may be erroneous in these and like studies.

In order to appreciate the actual outcomes implications of VTE in the ICU, clinicians must understand how the risk to benefit ratio for pharmacologic prophylaxis alters rates of bleeding in critically ill subjects. For example, an agent may prove extremely effective at prevention but lead to unacceptable rates of bleeding that undermine the value of the agent as an alternative for prevention. This is particularly true for prophylactic choices that are renally cleared. Approximately 20% of those admitted to a critical care unit have acute renal impairment due to either age, comorbid conditions (eg, hypertension, diabetes), or because of the acute disease requiring ICU level of care (eg, sepsis, acute myocardial infarction). Historically, some have expressed concern regarding the use of LMWHs because of the fact that they are renally metabolized. However, recent data suggests that LWMHs are generally safe in the ICU and do not elevate the risk for bleeding. Specifically, the Dalteparin's Influence on the Renally Compromised: Anti-Xa (DIRECT) study[28] enrolled 156 critically ill patients with severe renal insufficiency, defined as a creatinine clearance of less than 30 mL/min based on the Cockcroft Gault formula. These subjects received dalteparin 5000 IU once daily for DVT prophylaxis to assess if LMWH contributed significantly to bleeding in the setting of renal failure. The bioaccumulation (excess anticoagulation effect) of dalteparin was gauged using serial trough anti-Xa levels, which were drawn twice weekly. The definition for bioaccumulation was at least one trough anti-Xa level greater than 0.40 IU/mL. This threshold was selected because prior studies found that the risk of bleeding increases with levels greater than 0.40 IU/mL; trough levels between 0.10 and 0.40 IU/mL are considered a safe level of anticoagulation. Major bleeding served as the primary outcome measure, which was classified as one or more of the following: (1) a decrease in hemoglobin level of 2 g/dL or greater, (2) need for transfusion of 2 units of red cells or more without an increase in hemoglobin level, (3) a spontaneous decreases in systolic blood pressure of 20 mm Hg or greater or an increase in heart rate of 20 beats/min or greater or a decrease in systolic blood pressure of 10 mm Hg or greater while the patient was upright in the absence of another cause of hypotension,

(4) bleeding at a critical site, such as intracranial bleeding, or (5) bleeding at a wound site that required an intervention. The mean creatinine clearance in the cohort was 18.9 mL/min and the peak anti-Xa levels were between 0.29 and 0.34 IU/mL. The trough anti-Xa levels were undetectable (<0.10 IU/mL) or minimal (0.10 to 0.20 IU/mL) in 99% of the measurements. Only 10 patients (7.2%; 95% CI, 4.0% to 12.8%) had major bleeding, but there was no association between major bleeding and anti-Xa levels. Also, serial bilateral lower limb venous ultrasonography was performed within 48 hours of ICU admission and twice weekly thereafter. Similar to prior studies, the incidence of DVT was 5.1% (95% CI, 2.5% to 10.2%). Therefore, LMWH for DVT prophylaxis is safe and does not significantly influence bleeding risk in critically ill patients who have severe impairment in renal function.

In fact, the results from DIRECT and similar analyses suggest that the current anticoagulant dose used to prevent DVT in the ICU may be inadequate. In a small prospective observational study, anti-Xa levels were drawn in 45 patients (15 ICU patients on pressors, 15 ICU patients not on pressors, and 15 general surgical patients) patients who received nadoparin 2850 IU/day.[29] The anti-Xa levels of those in the ICU who required vasopressors was significantly lower than those in the other groups In another evaluation, anti-Xa levels were compared between 13 ward patients and 15 ICU patients who received enoxaparin 40 mg once daily for thromboprophylaxis. Again, the anti-Xa levels were significantly lower in the ICU patient.[30] There is uncertainty as to whether the use of vasopressors and/or the presence of generalized edema alters drug absorption, as both factors can affect drug uptake due to decreased subcutaneous perfusion.[31–33] Nevertheless, due to the small sample size of these studies, the impact of these observations is at best suggestive and hypothesis generating.

Those who have a contraindication to bleeding yet have a high risk for the development of VTE should receive mechanical VTE prophylaxis. Individuals who are actively bleeding, are considered too high risk for bleeding, or have profound thrombocytopenia should be considered for mechanical thromboprophylaxis. Unfortunately, the lack of a formal risk stratification tool to assist clinicians in objectively quantifying the risk for bleeding or the potential tolerability of VTE prophylaxis leaves clinicians weighing the risk:benefit ratio without clear guidance. Due to the paucity of evidence demonstrating the safety and efficacy of mechanical VTE prophylaxis and the high risk for VTE in the critical care population, transition to chemical thromboprophylaxis from mechanical modalities should be expedited when contraindications to its use resolve. Since a good portion of VTEs occur within the first week of admission to the ICU, those initially treated with mechanical VTE prophylaxis should be reassessed frequently for pharmacologic agents.

Currently, the ACCP recommends the use of UFH or LMWH for DVT prevention in the ICU. However, with the findings from PROTECT, these prevention guidelines may be modified. The lower PE rates in those who received LMWH may be significant enough to alter the practice of VTE prophylaxis in the ICU especially since PEs are less tolerable. The potential hemodynamic and respiratory deterioration associated with PE in the ICU is enough to warrant preferentially using LMWH for DVT prophylaxis when chemical agents are being considered. Unfortunately, PROTECT did not provide data on the mortality attributed to these higher rates of PE as it was not powered to address this issue. However, overall, there was no mortality difference between LMWH and UFH in PROTECT. Regardless, the ACCP guidelines strongly recommend the use of VTE prophylaxis in all critically ill patients. The use of chemical thromboprophylaxis is graded 1A in the guidelines indicating that high quality evidence exists to support its use in ICU patients. The use of mechanical thromboprophylaxis is only graded 1C because it is only recommended when chemical prophylaxis is not an option, but the evidence as to its efficacy is lacking.[26,34] Frequently in clinical practice, both chemical and mechanical modalities for prophylactic therapy are prescribed. Although there is no evidence that dual therapy is effective, the risks associated with this concomitant approach are minimal. Most important is the initiation of chemical anticoagulants, whether with or without mechanical modalities, when the risk of bleeding is low. Given these recommendations and the burden of illness related to VTE in the ICU, DVT prophylaxis should be assessed for and prescribed as soon as possible.

VTE PROPHYLAXIS HEALTH CARE POLICY

The growing evidence surrounding the safety and efficacy of VTE prophylaxis in both the ICU and general medical patients has caused the Centers for Medicare and Medicaid Services (CMS) to institute a policy mandating clinicians as well as hospital administration to carefully consider the systematic use of VTE prophylaxis. In an attempt to financially incentivize hospitals to improve quality of care, CMS is no longer willing to reimburse hospitals for the care of patients who develop a hospital-acquired VTE. Under the hospital inpatient prospective payment system (IPPS), this policy includes making hospitals assume the increased costs of managing conditions acquired during hospitalization that are deemed "reasonably preventable through adherence to evidence based guidelines." This policy is a logical extension of earlier CMS quality measures in surgery where CMS audits the use of peri- and postoperative DVT prevention as part of the Surgical Care Improvement Program (SCIP). The effectiveness of these rules in the surgical population has resulted in the extension of this CMS policy to the ICU patient. Additionally, CMS requires hospitals to report quality measures, such as use of VTE prophylaxis after surgery or in the ICU, contraindications to patient receiving VTE prophylaxis, and the incidence of VTE. Failure to comply with these enhanced reporting requirements leads to reductions in reimbursements. Therefore, vigilance to participate in the prevention of VTE in hospitalized patients is ever more important, as cumulative costs associated with VTE can be quite expensive. Hopefully, if the direct complications of VTE and the potential for mortality related to PE fail to motivate change in practice, the financial ramifications will motivate both institutional and provider behavior to change. Again, this evolution in financial systems underscores the need for all to be familiar with the most recent guidelines for VTE prevention.

ECONOMIC BURDEN OF VTE

In order to fully comprehend the impact of VTE as a healthcare burden, one must understand the costs associated with VTE. In the general medical population, estimates suggest that the cost of developing an inpatient DVT or PE adds $8,000 and $14,000, respectively to the entire hospital bill. The additional cumulative costs are even more impressive in those who develop both a DVT and PE simultaneously: approximately $28,000 per case.[35]

Yet, these figures are misleading and probably underestimate the true cost associated with the development of VTE. First, these estimates are only available for the general medical patient, and second, these estimates only reflect the short-term inpatient costs of VTE and hence are not comprehensive. Management of VTE is associated other potentially hidden costs. For example, after the initial VTE even, approximately 5% of patients will be readmitted to the hospital within 1 year.[35] These costs do not account for these readmissions and perhaps more concerning, some of these later sequelae of VTE are more costly and more devastating than the initial event. Select patients suffer from late, significant bleeding complications due to anticoagulant therapy, recurrent VTE, or other complications (ie, persistent pulmonary hypertension, post-thrombotic syndrome, chronic venous stasis). The costs associated with these readmissions for these reasons can often be higher than costs for the initial event: $11,862 for DVT and $14,722 for PE.[35] Furthermore, these figures are estimated costs for VTE in general medical patients but not for VTEs acquired in the sicker ICU patient population. Hence, these costs are an underestimate of costs associated with VTE in the critically ill.

One area of relative certainty is that patients with critical illness who develop VTE have longer ICU and hospital lengths of stay. This, too, contributes significantly to hospital costs, morbidity, and mortality. Illustrating this, patients who develop a VTE after major orthopedic surgery (total hip replacement, total knee replacement, or hip fracture repair) remain in the ICU longer than their counterparts who do not suffer a VTE. Comparatively, once a VTE occurs, the average ICU length of stay increases from 1 to 4 more days. These extra ICU days are associated with significantly higher hospital costs. Factors that can contribute to these increased costs include differences in the nurse:patient ratio, the equipment required for life-sustaining measures, and the need for closer monitoring. In fact, critically ill orthopedic patients who develop a DVT incur further costs of $17,114 and $18,521 for PE[36] compared to counterparts who never develop a VTE.

The key driver of increased costs related to VTE in the ICU is the effect that this condition has upon length of stay. For example, in a retrospective cohort study, ICU patients diagnosed with DVT had a median ICU length of stay of 7 days and 5 days for those diagnosed with a PE. Similarly, in another prospective observation study, the length of ICU stay and hospital stay both concomitantly increased when patients were diagnosed with VTE.[37] Those who experienced an in-hospital DVT spent 15.5 days in the ICU compared to only 9 days for those who did not develop DVT in the ICU ($P = .005$). Hospital length of stay also doubled from 23 to 51 days ($P<.001$) in the presence of a DVT[21]. Hence, VTE in critical care patients can result in significant morbidity and mortality as well as hospital costs.

These high costs associated with VTE acquired in the ICU may help influence the choice of an appropriate agent for chemical thromboprophylaxis. In general, given the economic implications of VTE in the ICU, any systematic approach to prevention will likely prove cost-effective if not cost saving. Specifically, the key issues affecting decisions about the cost-effectiveness of various options for thromboprophylaxis in the ICU focus on the efficacy of the alternative available, their relative safety, and the costs of the agents and the relative outcomes. It is crucial to appreciate that acquisition costs alone do not and cannot drive the decision about what types of agents to employ for VTE prevention. In light of the costs of VTE in the ICU, the greater expense of a novel agent relative to generic UFH may be well outweighed by either improved effectiveness or enhanced safety. In other words, the costs of the VTE and the bleeding tend to be the key determinants of cost-effectiveness in this situation. This was illustrated by Shorr and Ramage in a decision analysis involving trauma subjects. Despite the higher immediate costs associated with the administration of LMWH, they determined that the overall cost of using LMWH was about $28,000 less than UFH due to its better efficacy at preventing VTE in trauma patients. This point was also demonstrated in a meta-analysis evaluating the efficacy and safety of LMWH vs UFH in ischemic stroke. When pooling 3 RCTs, totaling 2024 stroke patients, LMWH significantly reduced VTE occurrence compared to UFH (OR, 0.54; 95% CI, 0.41 to 0.70; $P<.001$)[38] without increasing the risk for adverse events: intracranial hemorrhage (OR with LMWH, 0.75; 95% CI, 0.21 to 1.91; $P = .567$), major bleeding (OR with LMWH, 1.75; 95% CI, 0.73 to 4.20; $P = .551$), or overall mortality (OR with LMWH, 0.97; 95% CI, 0.69 to 1.33; $P = .633$). Surely, the improved effectiveness of LMWH is also more cost effective than UFH in this scenario. Findings from PROTECT, thus, beg for a formal cost-effectiveness analysis. Certainly, LMWHs, even if generic, cost more to purchase than do UFHs. Additionally, the overall similar efficacy and safety of dalteparin and UFH suggest that UFH may be preferred on economic ground. However, that fewer PEs occurred with the LMWH allow one to posit that dalteparin might be the cost-effective alternative. Given the costs of treating PE in the ICU, the central question becomes whether there was a difference in some measure of resource use (eg, length of stay, hospital costs, etc) in terms of lower rate of PEs associated with LMWH. Unfortunately, the initial PROTECT report sheds no light on this question. If there was no difference in length of stay or costs in the overall cohort then UFHs will likely prove the cost-effective strategy. If the converse is true, then LMWHs may be both clinically and economically superior in the ICU. We simply have insufficient data for answering this conundrum at present. As was mentioned above, UFH in PROTECT was administered only twice daily. Therefore any financial assessment of TID UFH cannot be accomplished with the results from PROTECT. Finally, current cost estimates do not account for pharmacy costs that can exceed $3000, outpatient pharmacy costs, and outpatient physician visits that are substantial. Thus, hospital acquired VTE is a considerable drain on resources. Clearly, given these direct and indirect costs, any systematic strategy to prevent the occurrence of VTE will be cost effective if not cost saving.

SUMMARY

Critically ill patients clearly face an increased risk for developing VTE. Upon admission, all critical care patients should be immediately assessed for and prescribed VTE prophylaxis as it can significantly reduce VTE occurrence, its potential sequelae, and costs associated with VTE treatment. The financial burden associated with VTE is substantial. Longer ICU and hospital lengths of stay, pharmacy costs, and further outpatient management all contribute considerably to the economic burden of disease. In addition, however, the policy of CMS to improve quality of care and withhold reimbursement for hospital-acquired illness will affect an individual hospital's functional capacity. Thus, from a safety and cost standpoint, the ACCP (8th edition) guidelines recommend the use of LMWH or UFH to prevent VTE in critical care patients. When chemical thromboprophylaxis is contraindicated, mechanical prophylaxis should be used until any potential contraindications resolve, at which point chemical prophylaxis should be initiated. The importance of this healthcare issue should motivate hospital administration and physicians to systematically initiate thromboprophylaxis in all ICU patients.

REFERENCES

1. Attia J, Ray JG, Cook DJ, et al. Deep vein thrombosis and its prevention in critically ill adults. Arch Intern Med 2001;161:1268–79.
2. Cade JF. High risk of the critically ill for venous thromboembolism. Crit Care Med 1982;10:448–50.
3. Fraisse F, Holzapfel L, Couland JM, et al. Nadroparin in the prevention of deep vein thrombosis in acute decompensated COPD. The Association of Non-University Affiliated Intensive Care Specialist Physicians of France. Am J Respir Crit Care Med 2000;161:1109–14.

4. McCarthy ST, Turner JJ, Robertson D, et al. Low-dose heparin as a prophylaxis against deep-vein thrombosis after acute stroke. Lancet 1977;2:800–1.

5. Kelly J, Rudd A, Lewis R, et al. Venous thromboembolism after acute stroke. Stroke 2001;32:262–7.

6. McCarthy ST, Turner J. Low-dose subcutaneous heparin in the prevention of deep-vein thrombosis and pulmonary emboli following acute stroke. Age Ageing 1986;15: 84–8.

7. Crowther MA, Cook DJ, Griffith LE, et al. Deep venous thrombosis: clinically silent in the intensive care unit. J Crit Care 2005;20:334–40.

8. Chan CM, Shorr AF. Venous thromboembolic disease in the intensive care unit. Semin Respir Crit Care Med 2010;31:39–46.

9. Dalen JE. Pulmonary embolism: what have we learned since Virchow? Natural history, pathophysiology, and diagnosis. Chest 2002;122:1440–56.

10. Kearon C. Natural history of venous thromboembolism. Circulation 2003;107(23 Suppl 1):I22–30.

11. Tapson VF. Acute pulmonary embolism. N Engl J Med 2008;358:1037–52.

12. Moser KM, LeMoine JR, Nachtwey FJ, et al. Deep venous thrombosis and pulmonary embolism. Frequency in a respiratory intensive care unit. JAMA 1981;246:1422–4.

13. Neuhaus A, Bentz RR, Weg JG. Pulmonary embolism in respiratory failure. Chest 1978;73:460–5.

14. Pingleton SK, Bone RC, Pingleton WW, et al. Prevention of pulmonary emboli in a respiratory intensive care unit: efficacy of low-dose heparin. Chest 1981;79:647–50.

15. Cullen DJ, Nemeskal AR. The autopsy incidence of acute pulmonary embolism in critically ill surgical patients. Intensive Care Med 1986;12:399–403.

16. Blosser SA, Zimmerman HE, Stauffer JL. Do autopsies of critically ill patients reveal important findings that were clinically undetected? Crit Care Med 1998;26:1332–6.

17. Geerts W, Cook D, Selby R, et al. Venous thromboembolism and its prevention in critical care. J Crit Care 2002;17:95–104.

18. Perkins GD, McAuley DF, Davies S, et al. Discrepancies between clinical and post-mortem diagnoses in critically ill patients: an observational study. Crit Care (Lond Engl) 2003;7:R129–32.

19. Fernandez-Segoviano P, Lazaro A, Esteban A, et al. Autopsy as quality assurance in the intensive care unit. Crit Care Med 1988;16:683–5.

20. Mort TC, Yeston NS. The relationship of pre mortem diagnoses and post mortem findings in a surgical intensive care unit. Crit Care Med 1999;27:299–303.

21. Cook D, Crowther M, Meade M, et al. Deep venous thrombosis in medical-surgical critically ill patients: prevalence, incidence, and risk factors. Crit Care Med 2005;33: 1565–71.

22. Ibrahim EH, Iregui M, Prentice D, et al. Deep vein thrombosis during prolonged mechanical ventilation despite prophylaxis. Crit Care Med 2002;30:771–4.

23. Samama MM, Cohen AT, Darmon JY, et al. A comparison of enoxaparin with placebo for the prevention of venous thromboembolism in acutely ill medical patients. Prophylaxis in Medical Patients with Enoxaparin Study Group. N Engl J Med 1999;341:793–800.

24. Leizorovicz A, Cohen AT, Turpie AG, et al. Randomized, placebo-controlled trial of dalteparin for the prevention of venous thromboembolism in acutely ill medical patients. Circulation 2004;110:874–9.

25. Cohen AT, Davidson BL, Gallus AS, et al. Efficacy and safety of fondaparinux for the prevention of venous thromboembolism in older acute medical patients: randomised placebo controlled trial. BMJ (Clin Res Ed) 2006;332(7537):325–9.

26. Geerts WH, Bergqvist D, Pineo GF, et al. Prevention of venous thromboembolism: American College of Chest Physicians Evidence-Based Clinical Practice Guidelines (8th Edition). Chest 2008;133(6 Suppl):381S–453S.

27. Cook D, Meade M, Guyatt G, et al. Dalteparin versus unfractionated heparin in critically ill patients. N Engl J Med 2011;364:1305–14.

28. Douketis J, Cook D, Meade M, et al. Prophylaxis against deep vein thrombosis in critically ill patients with severe renal insufficiency with the low-molecular-weight heparin dalteparin: an assessment of safety and pharmacodynamics: the DIRECT study. Arch Intern Med 2008;168:1805–12.

29. Dorffler-Melly J, de Jonge E, Pont AC, et al. Bioavailability of subcutaneous low-molecular-weight heparin to patients on vasopressors. Lancet 2002;359:849–50.

30. Priglinger U, Delle Karth G, Geppert A, et al. Prophylactic anticoagulation with enoxaparin: Is the subcutaneous route appropriate in the critically ill? Crit Care Med 2003;31:1405–9.

31. Haas CE, Kaufman DC, Jones CE, et al. Cytochrome P450 3A4 activity after surgical stress. Crit Care Med 2003;31:1338–46.

32. Jochberger S, Mayr V, Luckner G, et al. Antifactor Xa activity in critically ill patients receiving antithrombotic prophylaxis with standard dosages of certoparin: a prospective, clinical study. Crit Care (Lond Engl) 2005;9:R541–8.

33. Rommers MK, Van der Lely N, Egberts TC, et al. Anti-Xa activity after subcutaneous administration of dalteparin in ICU patients with and without subcutaneous oedema: a pilot study. Crit Care (Lond Engl) 2006;10:R93.

34. Guyatt GH, Cook DJ, Jaeschke R, et al. Grades of recommendation for antithrombotic agents: American College of Chest Physicians Evidence-Based Clinical Practice Guidelines (8th Edition). Chest 2008;133(6 Suppl):123S–31S.

35. Spyropoulos AC, Lin J. Direct medical costs of venous thromboembolism and subsequent hospital readmission rates: an administrative claims analysis from 30 managed care organizations. J Manag Care Pharm 2007;13:475–86.

36. Ollendorf DA, Vera-Llonch M, Oster G. Cost of venous thromboembolism following major orthopedic surgery in hospitalized patients. Am J Health Syst Pharm 2002;59:1750–4.

37. Patel R, Cook DJ, Meade MO, et al. Burden of illness in venous thromboembolism in critical care: a multicenter observational study. J Crit Care 2005;20:341–7.

38. Shorr AF, Jackson WL, Sherner JH, et al. Differences between low-molecular-weight and unfractionated heparin for venous thromboembolism prevention following ischemic stroke: a metaanalysis. Chest 2008;133:149–55.

Health Economics and Health Technology Assessment: Perspectives from Australia and New Zealand

Stephen Streat, MB, ChB, FRACP[a],*, Stephen Munn, MB, ChB, FRACS[b]

KEYWORDS

• Health economics • Health technology assessment
• Cost-effectiveness • Cost-utility analysis

Formal health economics and health technology assessment (HTA) processes, including cost-effectiveness and cost-utility analysis, are variably used to inform decisions about public and private health service funding and service provision. In general, pharmaceuticals have been subject to more sophisticated health economic analyses and HTAs and for a longer time than either devices or procedures. HTA has been performed by a number of different entities including agencies located within various government departments, private sector agencies, and academic and professional groups. While HTA shares many common features across the world, its uses, approaches, applications, and impact differ throughout the world. This chapter will discuss some of the general attributes of HTA and will focus on its specifiic applications in Australia and New Zealand. Australia and New Zealand (combined population 27 million) share similar cultural, economic, and political attributes. Both countries provide universal health care coverage within public health systems that combine taxation-based government financing with service provision by state-owned health care providers. Both countries also have private sector health service providers with a mixture of public and private (insurance-based and self-pay) financing. Australia spends about 25% more on health care per capita (at purchasing power parity) than does New Zealand and also provides a 30% taxation rebate to incentivize private health insurance. Both countries have similar regulatory frameworks for the

[a] Department of Critical Care Medicine, Auckland District Health Board, 2 Park Road, Grafton, Auckland 1023, New Zealand
[b] New Zealand Liver Transplant Unit, Auckland District Health Board, 2 Park Road, Grafton, Auckland 1023, New Zealand
* Corresponding author.
E-mail address: stephens@adhb.govt.nz

Crit Care Clin 28 (2012) 125–133
doi:10.1016/j.ccc.2011.10.008
0749-0704/12/$ – see front matter © 2012 Elsevier Inc. All rights reserved.

use of pharmaceuticals and medical devices and are working to establish common processes for their regulation. Although there are similarities in the processes used in both countries to assess pharmaceuticals, devices and services including procedures, in New Zealand the responsibility for assessment of pharmaceuticals has been combined with that of managing (including purchasing) pharmaceuticals within a capped budget and has been vested in a single government agency (PHARMAC), which will soon also be responsible for similar management of medical devices. This agency is under some potential threat as a result of ongoing trade negotiations with the United States. A recent Australian government review of HTA has initiated a large number of changes in the way that HTA is used there to inform decision-making. It is likely that HTA processes in both countries will become more aligned in future as part of the continued evolution of the close economic relationship between them.

HEALTH TECHNOLOGY ASSESSMENT DEFINED

HTA according to the International Society of Technology Assessment in Health Care, is the "systematic evaluation of the properties, effects and/or other impacts of health care technology."[1] The primary purpose of HTA is to provide organized and objective scientific, medical, health economic, and outcomes-based evidence to support clinicians, administrators, public health professionals, regulatory officials, and policymakers alike in decisions related to use and recommendations regarding drugs, diagnostics, devices, and other health care programs, techniques, and interventions.[1] HTAs are increasingly being used by governments, regulatory bodies, payers, and other agencies and organizations across the world, although their uses, applications, and impact vary in different countries and even different regions. While the discussion that follows focuses on Australia and New Zealand, the basic tenets of HTA are relatively similar.

AUSTRALIA AND NEW ZEALAND

Australia is a large continent (7.6 million square kilometers) in the Southwest Pacific with an estimated population of 22.6 million[2] in June 2011. The population is predominantly (about 90%) European, with about 8% being Asian and about 2% being Aboriginal or Torres Strait Islanders—the indigenous peoples of Australia. Australia ranks highly internationally on many measures of quality of life including educational attainment, economic, political, and press freedom and lack of corruption. It was ranked second in the world in 2010 (behind Norway) by the UN Development Programme[3] on the Human Development Index—a composite index of life expectancy, education, and income. Per capita GDP at purchasing power parity (PPP) was $39,406 in 2010, or 83% of US per capita GDP.[4] Total health expenditure per capita at PPP was $3445 in 2008,[5] similar to that of Canada and most of western Europe but less than half of U.S. health expenditure at PPP in 2008 ($7720).

New Zealand is a small (268,000 square kilometers) island nation in the South Pacific (estimated population about 4.4 million in June 2011) located about 2000 km from its nearest neighbors: Australia and other South Pacific island nations. The population is increasingly ethnically diverse, including about 15% who identify as Maori (the indigenous people) and about 15% as Asian or Pacific peoples.[6] New Zealand ranks similarly to Australia on many measures of quality of life including educational attainment, economic, political and press freedom and lack of corruption. It was ranked third in the world in 2010 (between Australia and the United States) by the UN Development Programme[3] on the Human Development Index. Per capita GDP at purchasing power parity (PPP) was $29,803 in 2010, or 63% of US per capita

GDP.[3] Total health expenditure per capita at PPP was $2784 in 2008,[5] around 80% of Australian expenditure and just over a third of US expenditure.

Australia and New Zealand (often collectively referred to as "Australasia"), share many similar national characteristics and have very close historical, cultural, and economic ties. There has been a free trade agreement between the two countries since 1965, which was made closer in 1983 and resulted in essentially free movement of goods and services by 1990. There has been free movement of people between the two countries since 1973 and there are substantial populations of each country's citizens in the other country. The governments of both countries are working to more closely harmonize regulatory agencies, including in health. Nevertheless, there are significant differences in wealth, history, culture, and politics, which are reflected in the differences in the health systems of the two countries.

OVERVIEW OF THE AUSTRALIAN AND NEW ZEALAND HEALTH SYSTEMS

Both countries provide universal health care coverage within public health systems, which combines taxation-based government financing and service provision by state-owned health care providers. Both countries also have private sector health service providers with a mixture of public and private (insurance-based and self-pay) financing. Australia provides a 30% taxation rebate to incentivise private health insurance. Government funding covered 65.4% of Australia's and 80.2% of New Zealand's health care expenditures in 2008.[7] National health care policies and regulation are the responsibilities of each government but there is increasing harmonisation of national standards and some regulatory mechanisms as part of the close economic relationship. Specialist medical colleges are binational and most national professional qualifications are recognised in both countries. Intensive care services in the two countries are generally similar in philosophy, structure and clinical practice but there are both more available intensive care beds (8.0 vs 4.8 per 100,000 population) and a higher proportion of private intensive care beds (30% vs 5%) in Australia.[8]

HEALTH ECONOMICS AND HEALTH TECHNOLOGY ASSESSMENT IN AUSTRALIA AND NEW ZEALAND

The development of health economics and HTA in both countries has been influenced strongly by the linkages between regulation, health care funding (especially public funding), and the purchasing of pharmaceuticals, devices, and specific health care services.

Regulation is an overarching government function and is primarily but not exclusively concerned with the protection of public health and safety. In Australia, the Therapeutic Goods Administration (TGA) is responsible for regulating both is medicines and medical devices, including that they "meet acceptable standards of quality, safety and efficacy (performance), when necessary" and ensuring that "the benefits to consumers outweigh any risks associated with the use of medicines and medical devices."[9] Similar functions in New Zealand are performed by the New Zealand Medicines and Medical Devices Safety Authority (Medsafe, http://www.medsafe. govt.nz/). This agency has historically focussed on medicines, rather than devices, but is currently updating its regulatory guidelines and codes. Evidence of safety (and not robust evidence of clinical efficacy) is required for medical devices to be registered and thus marketed within New Zealand. On June 20, 2011, the Prime Ministers of New Zealand and Australia announced that the New Zealand and Australian governments have agreed to proceed with a joint scheme for the regulation of therapeutic goods (medicines, medical devices, and biologicals). The joint arrangements will be administered by a single regulatory agency, the Australia New Zealand Therapeutic

Products Agency (ANZTPA), which will absorb the current regulators—Australia's TGA and New Zealand's Medsafe.

In response to a review of HTA in Australia[10] in 2009, the Australian federal Department of Health and Ageing developed a website (http://www.health.gov.au/hta) to provide an overview of HTA processes used to inform decisions about the registration of health technologies and the reimbursement of these technologies provided under various public and private funding arrangements. Included in recommendations from the review is recognition of a need for a national approach to HTA processes. Extensive restructuring of agencies and processes is under way, and signaled changes are expected to take place over the next 2 years or so in the way in which devices and services (including so-called co-dependent and hybrid technologies) are assessed.

PHARMACEUTICALS

The Australian Pharmaceutical Benefits Scheme (PBS) provides publically subsidised prescription medicines. The PBS is available to all Australian (and New Zealand) citizens, and residents of Australia with a permanent visa, as well as to visitors from countries (currently including Italy, New Zealand, the Republic of Ireland, Finland, Malta, the Netherlands, Sweden, Norway, the United Kingdom, and Belgium) with which Australia has a Reciprocal Health Care Agreement. A patient co-payment is usually required. This will be up to a maximum of $AUD34.20 ($USD35.75), or up to $AUD5.60 ($USD5.85) for holders of concession cards, such as the elderly. Pharmaceuticals can only be listed on the PBS after review and positive recommendation by the Pharmaceutical Benefits Advisory Committee (PBAC; http://www.pbs.gov.au/info/industry/listing/participants/pbac). This is an independent committee of medical and other health professionals, health economists, and consumer representatives appointed by the Australian government, which is required by legislation to consider both the effectiveness and cost of a proposed pharmaceutical compared to alternatives. PBAC includes an economics subcommittee that reviews and interprets economic analyses of pharmaceuticals. The primary focus of this analysis is the incremental cost-effectiveness of the proposed pharmaceutical including the costs associated with pharmaceuticals and other related health care resources and outcomes in terms of quality and length of life over a period of follow-up expected to cover any incremental (beneficial or adverse) effects and costs. PBAC also considers a number of other factors (including for example equity, affordability to the patient in the absence of subsidy and the anticipated cost via the PBS to the Australian government). The information required by PBAC is detailed, extensive, and comprehensive.[11] PBAC provides advice to the Pharmaceutical Benefits Pricing Authority (PBPA) about PBS listing, including advice about possible restrictions on the indications where PBS subsidy is available, and about alternative pharmaceuticals and comparative cost-effectiveness. The detail of the PBAC review process contains, inter alia, commercially sensitive information and is not made public, but the review outcomes are made publically available in a generic reporting style, such as, "The PBAC deferred the application due to issues with regard to the economic evidence" or "The application was rejected because of insufficient demonstration of effectiveness across the full population of patients for whom listing is requested and unfavourable cost-effectiveness."[12] The Pharmaceutical Benefits Pricing Authority (PBFA)[13] considers the advice provided by PBAC, along with proposed price and overseas prices (commonly in the United Kingdom and New Zealand), alternatives listed on the PBS and their prices and estimates of the costs to the government of listing the pharmaceutical on the PBS. It also negotiates price if possible (including possible risk-sharing or rebate arrangements) with suppliers of potentially listed pharmaceuticals and recommends to the government a price that should be paid. The predicted net cost to the PBS is taken into account by the government when taking a decisions about listing the pharmaceutical and how much to pay for it. Although the cost to the government results directly from PBS listing and subsequent prescription of listed pharmaceuticals, the PBS budget is not explicitly capped. Should the responsible Minister determine that the pharmaceutical be listed and subsidised on the PBS, but agreement on price cannot be reached with the supplier, the patient must pay an additional co-payment (on top of the normal PBS co-payment). As a result of these processes, Australians enjoy largely affordable access to a wide range of effective pharmaceuticals, albeit often with a modest patient co-payment.

Similar assessment processes are used for pharmaceuticals in New Zealand. The New Zealand pharmaceutical management agency (PHARMAC; http://www.pharmac.govt.nz/) was established in 1993 with the statutory purpose to "secure for people in need of pharmaceuticals, the best health outcomes that are reasonably achievable from pharmaceutical treatment and from within the amount of funding provided." The activities of PHARMAC include deciding which pharmaceuticals are subsidised (and to what extent), negotiating (bulk, national) contracts with pharmaceutical suppliers *within a capped budget* for subsidised pharmaceuticals and also promoting the most effective use of pharmaceuticals to health professionals and the public. When deciding what pharmaceuticals are subsidised PHARMAC considers these nine criteria[14]:

1. The health needs of all eligible people within New Zealand
2. The particular health needs of Maori and Pacific peoples
3. The availability and suitability of existing medicines, therapeutic medical devices and related products and related things
4. The clinical benefits and risks of pharmaceuticals
5. The cost-effectiveness of meeting health needs by funding pharmaceuticals rather than using other publicly funded health and disability support services
6. The budgetary impact (in terms of the pharmaceutical budget and the government's overall health budget) of any changes to the schedule
7. The direct cost to health service users
8. The government's priorities for health funding, as set out in any objectives notified by the Crown to PHARMAC, or in PHARMAC's Funding Agreement, or elsewhere; and
9. Such other criteria as PHARMAC thinks fit. PHARMAC will carry out appropriate consultation when it intends to take any such "other criteria" into account.

PHARMACs economic analysis includes cost-utility analysis and what are termed "Technology Assessment Reports." The methodology used for cost-utility analysis is rigorous, has been peer-reviewed, and is publically available.[15] Most Technology Assessment Reports contain commercially sensitive information and are not published, but several have been made publicly available (eg, a review of COX-2 inhibitors[16] in 2003, at which time PHARMAC decided not to fund these agents). This example fortuitously gives an insight into some of the possible consequences of adding a novel pharmaceutical to a publically subsidized schedule without a funding cap. In Australia, COX-2 inhibitors were listed on the PBS in August 2000, with an expected first-year cost to government of about $AUD40m. However, the actual cost in the first year was over $AUD170m and this rose to $AUD218.6m by 2003.[15] COX-2 inhibitors were available but not subsidised in New Zealand over this time. PHARMAC estimated[17] that had New Zealand funded COX-2 inhibitors at the same time as Australia, this may have resulted in approximately 740 to 4220 excess myocardial infarctions and approximately 330 to 1900 excess deaths from myocardial infarction over 4 years (in a population of about 4 million at that time). Not funding these agents (estimated to cost $NZD30m per year) allowed PHARMAC to fund or extend access to at least 18 pharmaceutical treatments, including statins, alendronate, venlafaxine, leflunomide, newer antiepileptic agents, and olanzapine and was estimated to save 437 "statistical lives" per year (ie, if COX-2 inhibitors had been funded, then the equivalent of 437 lives would have been lost per year from not receiving other pharmaceutical treatments).[18]

In contrast to the situation in Australia and other countries with publicly subsidized pharmaceutical schedules, PHARMAC also purchases pharmaceuticals for New Zealand from within a capped budget set by the government. PHARMAC has been widely credited with substantial savings as a result of its assessment processes and purchasing arrangements, which include widespread use of generic pharmaceuticals and tough negotiating with suppliers. This process has resulted in generally affordable access to a similar wide range of effective pharmaceuticals being available in New Zealand as in Australia. However, New Zealand often has a more limited number of different of pharmaceuticals within classes and provides pharmaceuticals later than in Australia and with a small patient co-payment. (The schedule of subsidized pharmaceuticals is also searchable online at http://www.pharmac.govt.nz/healthpros/Schedule).

PHARMAC uses other criteria for funding in addition to a cost-utility measure and has recently refuted[19] the suggestion that there is a specific funding threshold (eg, in cost/QALY) for pharmaceuticals in New Zealand.[20] New Zealand and the United States are currently in negotiation over a closer trade relationship and PHARMAC has been identified in New Zealand[21] as a possible casualty of these negotiations following lobbying by the largely US-based pharmaceutical industry and representations to President Obama by 28 members of the US Congress.[22]

DEVICES AND SERVICES

HTA is used in Australia as part of decision-making about whether a particular health technology is reimbursed by public (government) or private (insurance) funders.

The Australian Medicare program provides access to medical and hospital services for all Australian residents and certain categories of visitors to Australia. The Medicare Benefits Schedule (MBS) is a listing of the Medicare services subsidised by the Australian government. Medicare benefits required to be paid (under legislation) are payable for professional services, defined as clinically relevant services listed in the MBS. A medical service is clinically relevant if it is generally accepted in the medical profession as necessary for the appropriate treatment of the patient. The Australian government uses a ministerially appointed committee, the Medical Services Advisory Committee (MSAC; http://www.msac.gov.au/), to assess new technologies that have been proposed to be added to the MBS. MSAC reviews the strength of the evidence relating to the safety, effectiveness, and cost-effectiveness of new medical technologies and procedures. MSAC conducts some HTA itself and has contracted some HTA to other agencies, in both Australia (eg, The Australian Safety and Efficacy Register of New Interventional Procedures–Surgical [ASERNIP-S]; http://www.surgeons.org/racs/research-and-audit/asernip-s, an endeavor of the Royal Australasian College of Surgeons) and New Zealand (see, for example, Cardiac resynchronisation therapy for severe heart failure[23]).

Following its review of the new technology, MSAC advises the Australian Minister for Health and Ageing of these matters. The decision about whether a relevant technology or procedure is listed in the MBS is made by the Minister, carrying with it the implication of public funding.

The Australian government is also involved in the assessment and listing of prostheses for private health insurance coverage. Private health insurers in Australia are required by legislation to pay benefits for a range of prostheses that are provided as part of an episode of hospital treatment for which a patient has insurance cover and for which a (government-funded) Medicare benefit is payable for the associated professional service. Such prostheses include cardiac pacemakers and defibrillators, cardiac stents, hip and knee replacements, and intraocular lenses, as well as human tissues such as human heart valves, corneas, bones, and muscle tissue.

However, when the Australian government is the funder of a particular health technology, the decision on funding is made in consideration of a number of factors other than HTA alone, including community opinion, the nature of the patient group affected, the impact of the disease in question, the availability of effective alternative treatments, and the total amount of funding for health care. Implementation of new technologies and services within Australia has largely taken place on a state rather than a national basis, which has resulted in some degree of inconsistency between states. Within local health areas, application of new technologies has been contained in various ways, including, for example, by providing them at certain hospitals only, or by limiting the number of procedures involving those technologies at those hospitals.

In New Zealand, there have not yet been analogous national HTA programs for publically funded devices and services although HTA reports have been prepared on a variety of specific topics by a number of independent agencies, such as New Zealand Health Technology Assessment (NZHTA; http://nzhta.chmeds.ac.nz/), which was a clearinghouse for HTA, which operated in New Zealand between 1997 and 2007, and Health Services Assessment Collaboration (http://www.healthsac.net/), which is a university-based research initiative. Recently, the New Zealand government has signaled an intention to broaden the scope of PHARMACs management responsibilities beyond pharmaceuticals to include medical devices.[24]

PHARMAC has previously only provided advice on a small number of medical devices to District Health Boards, which themselves were responsible for purchasing. Extension of the "PHARMAC model" to devices will require some legislative and other changes and the effects of this are yet to be seen.

There has not been a national and comprehensive HTA process for new services in New Zealand, although some ad hoc assessments have taken place; for example, the Auckland District Health Board maintains a clinical practice committee (of which the authors are members), which assesses new potential new services, including by cost-utility analysis. Recently reviewed services include, for example, transcatheter aortic valve implantation and renal denervation for refractory hypertension. Some of the recommendations of this committee have been used elsewhere in New Zealand to inform implementation decisions by other health funders and providers. Recently, a national health committee has been appointed by the government, which intends to use HTA processes in review of proposed new national and tertiary health services, obtaining HTA advice for this endeavour under contract from a variety of Australian and New Zealand agencies.

REFERENCES

1. Hailey D. Elements of Effectiveness for Health Technoloyg Assessment Programs. HTA Initiative #9, Alberta Heritage Foundation for Medical Research, Edmonton, Alberta, Canada, 2003. Available at: http://www.inahta.org/upload/HTA_resources/AboutHTA_Elements_of_Effectiveness_for_HTA_Programs.pdf. Accessed October 7, 2011.

2. Australia's population. Australian Bureau of Statistics. Available at: http://www.abs.gov.au/. Accessed June 10, 2011.

3. The Real Wealth of Nations: Pathways to Human Development. Human Development Report 2010. United Nations Development Programme, UN Plaza, New York, NY 10017, USA. Available at: http://hdr.undp.org/en/. Accessed November 16, 2010.

4. Organisation for Economic Cooperation and Development (OECD). Breakdown of Gross Domestic Product per capita in its components. Available at: http://stats.oecd.org/Index.aspx?DataSetCode=DECOMP. Accessed August 22, 2011.

5. Organisation for Economic Cooperation and Development (OECD). Health Expenditure and Financing. Available at: http://stats.oecd.org/. Accessed August 22, 2011.

6. New Zealand Census Data 2006. Statistics New Zealand, Wellington. Available at: http://www.stats.govt.nz/. Accessed August 20, 2011.

7. World Health Organisation. World Health Statistics 2011. Available at: http://www.who.int/entity/whosis/whostat/EN_WHS2011_Full.pdf. Accessed May 10, 2011.

8. Drennan K, Hart GK, Hicks P. Intensive Care Resources and Activity: Australia and New Zealand 2006/2007. ANZICS, Melbourne. 2008. Available at: http://www.anzics.com.au/. Accessed November 23, 2010.

9. Australian Government Department of Health and Ageing. Therapeutic Goods Administration. Australian regulatory guidelines for prescription medicines. 2004. Canberra, ACT. Available at: http://www.tga.gov.au/pdf/pm-argpm.pdf. Accessed July 10, 2011.

10. Australian Government Department of Health and Ageing. Review of Health Technology Assessment in Australia. Barton ACT, 2009. Available at: http://www.health.gov.au/internet/main/publishing.nsf/Content/00E847C9D69395B9CA25768F007F589A/$File/hta-review-report.pdf. Accessed July 10, 2011.

11. Australian Government Department of Health and Ageing Pharmaceutical Benefits Advisory Committee. Guidelines for preparing submissions to the Pharmaceutical Benefits Advisory Committee (Version 4.3), December 2008, Canberra ACT. Available at: http://www.pbs.gov.au/industry/listing/elements/pbacguidelines/PBAC4.3.2.pdf. Accessed July 10, 2011.

12. Commonwealth Department of Health and Ageing. Open letter to pharmaceutical companies. Available at: http://www.health.gov.au/internet/main/publishing.nsf/Content/86C324EA5E108324CA2572BA007D0197/$File/pbac_outcomes_info_letter.pdf. Accessed July 10, 2011.

13. Pharmaceutical Benefits Pricing Authority. Policies, procedures and methods used in the recommendations for pricing of pharmaceutical products. April 2009. Available at: http://www.health.gov.au/internet/main/publishing.nsf/Content/1D0AFBEEF35A185DCA2572B200015F5F/$File/PBPA-Manual-May%202009.pdf. Accessed July 10, 2011.

14. New Zealand Government Pharmaceutical Management Agency (PHARMAC). Decision criteria. May 8, 2009. Wellington. Available at: http://www.pharmac.govt.nz/patients/DecisionMakingProcess/DecisionCriteria. Accessed August 20, 2011.

15. New Zealand Government Pharmaceutical Management Agency (PHARMAC). Prescription for pharmacoeconomic analysis—methods for cost-utility analysis. May 2007, Wellington. Available at: http://www.pharmac.govt.nz/2007/06/19/PFPAFinal.pdf. Accessed August 20, 2011.

16. New Zealand Government Pharmaceutical Management Agency (PHARMAC). Celecoxib and rofecoxib—selective COX-2 inhibitors—for osteoarthritis and rheumatoid arthritis. 2003, Wellington. Available at: http://www.pharmac.govt.nz/2004/04/23/Cox2.pdf. Accessed August 20, 2011.

17. Grocott R, Metcalfe S. Going against the flow: the impact of PHARMAC not funding COX-2 inhibitors for chronic arthritis. N Z Med J 2005;118:1690.
18. New Zealand Government Pharmaceutical Management Agency (PHARMAC). New Zealand Pharmaceutical Schedule. August 2011, Wellington. Available at: http://www.pharmac.govt.nz/2011/07/27/Sched.pdf. Accessed August 20, 2011.
19. Metcalfe S, Grocott R. Comments on "Simoens, S. Health economic assessment: a methodological primer. Int. J. Environ. Res. Public Health 2009, 6, 2950–2966"— New Zealand in fact has no cost-effectiveness threshold. Int J Environ Res Public Health 2010;7:1831–4.
20. Simoens S. Health economic assessment: a methodological primer. Int J Environ Res Public Health 2009;6:2950–66.
21. Foster RH, Wilson N. Will Pharmac become a victim of its own success? BMJ 2011;2:d4908.
22. Moynihan R. New Zealand agency comes under pressure to pay more for drugs. BMJ. 2011;342:d3933.
23. Commonwealth of Australia. Cardiac resynchronisation therapy for severe heart failure. MSAC application 1042. 2005, Canberra. Available at: http://nzhta.chmeds.ac.nz/publications/crt_final.pdf. Accessed August 22, 2011.
24. Tony Ryall, Minister of Health, New Zealand Government. Government extends Pharmac role. Wellington, July 22, 2010. Available at: http://www.beehive.govt.nz/release/government-extends-pharmac-role. Accessed August 22, 2011.

Index

Note: Page numbers of article titles are in **boldface** type.

A

Acute kidney injury (AKI)
  in critically ill patients
    cardiac surgery–associated, 100
    contrast-induced nephropathy, 100–101
    described, 99–100
    economics of, 99–101
    outcomes of, 101
    RRT for
      financial aspects of, 104–105
  described, 99–100
  septic
    in critically ill patients, 100
Acute tubular necrosis (ATN)
  in critically ill patients
    treatment of
      economics of, 102–103
AKI. *See* Acute kidney injury (AKI)
Australia
  described, 126
  health care systems in
    overview of, 127
  health economics in, 127–128
    devices and services, 130–131
    pharmaceuticals-related, 128–130
  HTA in, 127–128
Australian Pharmaceutical Benefits Scheme (PBS), 128

B

Biomarkers
  in prediction of need for RRT and recovery chances, 107

C

CABG. *See* Coronary artery bypass graft (CABG)
Cardiac rehabilitation
  for cardiovascular disease in U.S., 82
Cardiovascular disease
  in U.S.
    cardiac rehabilitation for
      cost-effectiveness of, 82

Crit Care Clin 28 (2012) 135–141
doi:10.1016/S0749-0704(11)00102-3
0749-0704/12/$ – see front matter © 2012 Elsevier Inc. All rights reserved.

criticalcare.theclinics.com

economics of, **77–88**
 direct health care costs, 79–80
 discussion, 84–85
 indirect health care costs, 80
 limitations of, 80–81
epidemiology of, 78–79
ICD for
 cost-effectiveness of, 82
incidence of, 78
medical treatment for
 cost-effectiveness of, 81–83
  statins, 82
mortality data, 77, 78
prevalence of, 78
risk factors for, 78–79
surgical treatment for
 cost-effectiveness of, 83–84
Catheter-related bloodstream infection (CRBSI)
 in ICU
  prevention of
   economic aspects of, 89–90, 95
Congestive heart disease
 in U.S.
  medical treatment for
   cost-effectiveness of
    statins, 81–82
Continuous renal replacement therapy (CRRT)
 for ATN
  in critically ill patients
   economics of, 103
 SLEDD *vs.*
  in critically ill patients
   economics of, 105–106
Continuous renal replacement therapy (CRRT) program
 development of
  economics of, 106–107
Contrast-induced nephropathy
 AKI associated with
  in critically ill patients, 100–101
Coronary artery bypass graft (CABG)
 PCI *vs.*
  for cardiovascular disease in U.S.
   cost-effectiveness of, 83–84
Cost(s). *See specific topic*
Cost-benefit analysis
 in economic evaluation, 13
Cost-effectiveness analysis
 in economic evaluation, 12
Cost-minimization analysis
 in economic evaluation, 12
Cost-utility analysis
 in economic evaluation, 12–13

CRBSI. *See* Catheter-related bloodstream infection (CRBSI)
Critical care medicine
  costs of, **1–10**
    control strategies related to, 8
    data on, 2
    determination of, 1
    global approaches to
      limitations of, 8
    national hospital databases on, 2
    NHEs, 1
    in U.S.
      calculation of, 3
      studies of, 3–5
CRRT. *See* Continuous renal replacement therapy (CRRT)
Cystatin C
  in prediction of need for RRT and recovery chances, 107

D

Discounting, 16
Drotrecogin alfa
  in sepsis management
    cost-effectiveness analyses, 67

E

Economic(s). *See specific topic*
Economic evaluations
  health-related, **11–24**. *See also* Health economic methods

H

Health care
  costs of
    in U.S., 1
Health care system(s)
  in Australia and New Zealand, **125–133**. *See also* Australia; New Zealand
  costs within, 31–32
Health care–associated infections
  in ICU
    prevention of
      economic aspects of, **89–97**
        CRBSI, 89–90, 95
        VAP, 91–96
Health economic(s)
  assessment of
    perspectives from Australia and New Zealand, **125–133**
      devices and services, 130–131
      pharmaceuticals-related, 128–130
Health economic methods, **11–24**
  combining costs and outcomes, 16–18
  cost-benefit analysis, 13

cost-effectiveness analysis, 12
cost-minimization analysis, 12
cost-related measurements, 14–15
cost-utility analysis, 12–13
discounting, 16
modeled economic evaluations, 19–20
outcome-related measurements, 15–16
perspectives on, 13–14
results of
  use of, 22
trial-based economic evaluations, 18–19
types of, 11–13
uncertainty related to
  dealing with, 21–22
Health technology assessment (HTA)
  defined, 126
  perspectives from Australia and New Zealand, **125–133**
Heart surgery
  AKI associated with
    in critically ill patients, 100
Hemodialysis
  for ATN
    in critically ill patients
      economics of, 102
HTA. *See* Health technology assessment (HTA)

I

ICD. *See* Implantable cardioverter-defibrillator (ICD)
ICU. *See* Intensive care unit (ICU)
Implantable cardioverter-defibrillator (ICD)
  for cardiovascular disease in U.S., 82
Intensive care unit (ICU)
  costs within, 26–31
    decreasing length of stay–related, 26–27
    staffing, 27–30
      intensivist staffing, 28–29
      multidisciplinary teams, 29–30
      nursing, 28
    standardization of care–related, 30–31
  health care–associated infections in
    prevention of
      economic aspects of, **89–97**. *See also* Health care–associated infections, in
        ICU, prevention of, economic aspects of
  organization and management of
    economics of, **25–37**
      costs within healthcare system, 31–32
      fixed *vs.* variable costs, 26
      perspective regarding costs, 26
  VTE disease in, **113–123**. *See also* Venous thromboembolic (VTE) disease, in ICU

K

Kidney disease
in critically ill patients
economics of, **99–111**
AKI, 99–101
ATN, 102–103
evaluations related to
cost studies, 103–107
resources for, 103–107

L

Low tidal volume ventilation
cost-effectiveness of, 48

M

Mechanical ventilation
economics of, **39–55**
cost-effectiveness evaluation, 42–45
in critical care, 42
implications of literature, 45
incremental costs, 40–42
management strategies, 48–49
low tidal volume ventilation
cost-effectiveness of, 48
noninvasive
cost-effectiveness of, 49–50
economics of, 49–51
implications of literature, 50–51
outcomes of, 39–40
prolonged, 45–47
cost-effectiveness of, 45–47
economic burden of, 45
implications of literature, 47
Modeled economic evaluations, 19–20

N

National health expenditures (NHEs)
in U.S., 1
National hospital databases
on costs of critical care medicine, 2
Nephropathy
contrast-induced
AKI associated with
in critically ill patients, 100–101
Neutrophil gelatinase–associated lipocalin (NGAL)
in prediction of need for RRT and recovery chances, 107
New Zealand
described, 126–127
health care systems in
overview of, 127

health economics in, 127–128
  devices and services, 130–131
  pharmaceuticals-related, 128–130
HTA in, 127–128
NHEs. *See* National health expenditures (NHEs)

P

PBS. *See* Pharmaceutical Benefits Scheme (PBS)
PCI. *See* Percutaneous coronary intervention (PCI)
Percutaneous coronary intervention (PCI)
  CABG *vs.*
    for cardiovascular disease in U.S.
      cost-effectiveness of, 83–84
Pharmaceutical Benefits Scheme (PBS)
  Australian, 128

R

Renal failure
  in critically ill patients
    economics of, **99–111**
Renal replacement therapy (RRT)
  for AKI
    in critically ill patients
      economics of, 104–105
  need for
    prediction of
      biomarkers in, 107
Respiratory failure
  acute
    mechanical ventilation for, **39–55**
      cost-effectiveness of, 43–44
    economics of, **39–55**
      implications of literature, 45
    epidemiology of, 39–40
Russell equation
  alternative uses for, 5–8
  goal of, 3
  solving of
    approaches to, 5–8

S

Sepsis
  cost-effectiveness analyses in, 64–70
    drotrecogin alfa management, 67
    integrated sepsis protocols, 67–70
    nosocomial sepsis prevention strategies, 65–66
  defined, 57
  economics of, **57–76**
    costs
      burden of illness–related, 64
      international, 61

intrapathogenic variation in, 63–64
  sources of, 59–60
  in U.S., 60–61
epidemiology of, 58–59
nosocomial
  costs of, 62–63
  prevention strategies
    cost-effectiveness analyses in, 65–66
SLEDD. *See* Slow low-efficiency daily dialysis (SLEDD)
Slow low-efficiency daily dialysis (SLEDD)
  for ATN
    in critically ill patients
      economics of, 102–103
    CRRT *vs.*
      in critically ill patients
        economics of, 105–106
Statins
  for cardiovascular disease in U.S.
    cost-effectiveness of, 82
  for congestive heart disease in U.S.
    cost-effectiveness of, 81–82

T

Trial-based economic evaluations, 18–19

V

VAP. *See* Ventilator-associated pneumonia (VAP)
Venous thromboembolic (VTE) disease
  described, 113
  in ICU, **113–123**
    economic burden of, 119–121
    epidemiology of, 114–115
    outcomes aspects of, 119–121
    potentially devastating consequences of, 113–114
    prevention of, 115–119
      health care policy in, 119
    risk factors for, 115
Ventilation
  low tidal volume
    cost-effectiveness of, 48
  mechanical
    economics of, **39–55**. *See also* Mechanical ventilation, economics of
Ventilator-associated pneumonia (VAP)
  in ICU
    prevention of
      economic aspects of, 91–96
VTE disease. *See* Venous thromboembolic (VTE) disease

Moving?

Make sure your subscription moves with you!

To notify us of your new address, find your **Clinics Account Number** (located on your mailing label above your name), and contact customer service at:

Email: journalscustomerservice-usa@elsevier.com

800-654-2452 (subscribers in the U.S. & Canada)
314-447-8871 (subscribers outside of the U.S. & Canada)

Fax number: 314-447-8029

Elsevier Health Sciences Division
Subscription Customer Service
3251 Riverport Lane
Maryland Heights, MO 63043

*To ensure uninterrupted delivery of your subscription, please notify us at least 4 weeks in advance of move.

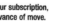

Printed and bound by CPI Group (UK) Ltd, Croydon, CR0 4YY

03/10/2024

01040456-0012

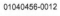